DR. BRADY'S

HEALTHY REVOLUTION

What You Really Need to Know to Stay Healthy in a Sick World

- Can't make sense of all those diet and alternative medicine books?

- Which diet books are right and which ones are wrong?

- Are vitamins and other supplements really necessary?

- Do safe natural alternatives for many common drugs really exist?

- Are herbs really safe and effective?

- What easy lifestyle changes can actually make a big difference in your health?

- Are there doctors and healthcare providers who really understand wellness and can help you?

- Is there an easy way to determine which foods and supplements you really need?

DR. DAVID M. BRADY

DR. BRADY'S
HEALTHY REVOLUTION

What You Really Need to Know to Stay Healthy in a Sick World

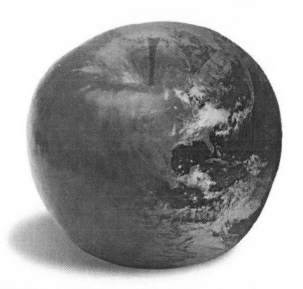

DR. DAVID M. BRADY

New York

Dr. Brady's
Healthy
Revolution

What You Really Need to Know
to Stay Healthy in a Sick World

by Dr. David M. Brady

© 2007 Dr. David M. Brady. All rights reserved.

ISBN: 978-1-60037-081-6 (Paperback)
ISBN: 978-1-60037-080-9 (Hardcover)
ISBN: 978-1-60037-082-3 (eBook)
ISBN: 978-1-60037-083-0 (Audio)

Published by:

MORGAN · JAMES™
THE ENTREPRENEURIAL PUBLISHER
www.morganjamespublishing.com

Morgan James Publishing, LLC

1225 Franklin Ave. Ste 325

Garden City, NY 11530-1693

Toll Free 800-485-4943

www.MorganJamesPublishing.com

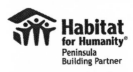

Habitat for Humanity®
Peninsula
Building Partner

Interior Design by:
Bonnie Bushman
bbushman@bresnan.net

Disclaimer

The material in this book is for informational purposes only and is not intended for the treatment or diagnosis of individual disease. Please visit a qualified medical or other health professional for specific diagnosis and treatment of any ailments mentioned or discussed in this book.

This book is not meant to serve as medical advice and should not be interpreted to replace the necessity for diagnosis and direct management by a qualified healthcare provider.

Dedication

This book is dedicated to my mentors, teachers, colleagues, patients, and friends who inspire me to think outside the lines and who motivate me to continue searching and seeking that which is wonderful about alternative, complementary, and integrative medicine. You know who you are. I thank you with all my heart.

Special Thanks

I would like to thank several individuals who have provided motivation, support and critique that greatly improved this book, including Roger Koehler, Jonathan & Linda Lizotte, Dr. Jeff Moss, J.J. Virgin, Steve Wickham and Stacey Brady. I also greatly appreciate the help I received in editing this manuscript by Susan Tafralis and, especially, the best teacher in California, Judy Sue Dixon.

Yours in wellness and vitality,

Dr. David M. Brady

About the Author
Dr. David M. Brady

Dr. Brady is a licensed Naturopathic Physician, a Board Certified Clinical Nutritionist, and a Diplomate of the American Clinical Board of Nutrition. He also completed an undergraduate degree in electrical engineering technology and was employed by McDonnell Douglas Aerospace Corporation before starting his clinical education. He is presently the *Director* of the *Human Nutrition Institute* at the University of Bridgeport and an *Associate Professor of Clinical Sciences* at the University of Bridgeport Colleges of Naturopathic Medicine and Chiropractic in Bridgeport, Connecticut. Dr. Brady is the *Chief Medical Officer* of Designs for Health, Inc., a nutriceutical and nutritional supplement manufacturer. He has been a leading nutritional product formulator and clinical consultant to some of the most innovative nutriceutical companies and clinical laboratories in the country during the past 15 years. Dr. Brady is a very popular lecturer and has appeared on speaking panels of numerous major scientific conferences in the field of nutritional and integrative medicine throughout the world. Dr. Brady maintains a private practice at *The Center for the Healing Arts* in Orange, CT where he specializes in *"Functional and Metabolic Medicine"*.

Dr. Brady lives in Connecticut with the loves of his life, his wife Stacey (a professional dance performer and dance instructor with the New England Ballet Company), his son Ian (a future center fielder for the New York Yankees), a new baby on the way, and his 1968 and 1969 Pontiac Firebirds.

HealthyRevolution.info
DrDavidBrady.com

Table of Contents

Introduction 1

Diet 7

Vitamins 39

Herbs 65

Lifestyles 99

Creating Your Unique Nutrition Program 121

    Comprehensive Metabolic Profiling 122

The Providers 127

    Medical & Osteopathic Physicians 127

    Chiropractic Physicians 130

    Naturopathic Physicians 135

    Herbalists 139

    Homeopaths 143

    Nutritionists & Dieticians 147

    Acupuncturists & Oriental Medicine 148

    Massage Therapist 153

    Esoteric and Intuitive Healers 156

The New Paradigm: "The New Medicine" 159

The Disorders 163

    ADHD 164

    Anxiety 165

    Arthritis 166

    Bladder Infection 168

Cold and Flu..168
Constipation 169
Depression...169
Diabetes...170
Diarrhea...172
Fibromyalgia 172
High Blood Pressure 174
High Cholesterol 175
Hypothyroid 176
Inflammation & Injury 177
Muscle Tightness & Spasm.................................178
Stress 178
Resources...181

Recommended Reading 181
Resources and Organizations..............................187
Accredited Naturopathic Medical Programs.........189
Naturopathic Licensure......................................190

Introduction

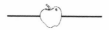

If you are like everyone else, you are confused by the myriad of diet, vitamin, herb, self-help and alternative therapy books available on the market these days. It seems as if every time you go to a bookstore or supermarket you see a new book that often contradicts what you have read in another book. Ten years ago you would have had to look long and hard to find one or two books with similar subject matter. Why are there so many new books on subjects such as these? The answer is simple. The public wants them! Authors are attempting to capitalize on the ever-increasing demand for answers and advice on how to live healthy and longer and comprehensive answers for many of these questions are often unavailable from family doctors.

The decade of the nineties brought a tidal wave of changes to the way medicine is practiced in the Western industrialized world. These changes created shock waves that have rattled the very foundation of standard medicine as we know it. For most of the twentieth century organized medicine influenced society far more than society influenced it. This all changed in the 1990's when an undercurrent of discontent with the standard allopathic model of healthcare reached a fevered pitch. Allopathic medicine is the type of conventional or standard medicine we have all become familiar with in Western countries. This system of medicine almost exclusively relies on drugs and surgery to relieve symptoms. Conventional allopathic medicine often places very little emphasis on altering lifestyles and diets of patients or in utilizing more natural, non-toxic treatments that are often available. Make no mistake about it, medicine is not changing willingly. It is being dragged kicking and screaming toward change by patients. Many believe that the straw that broke the camel's back was the advent of widespread managed care, or shall I say *managed inferior care*, during the 1980's. Several studies published in major family practice medical journals have shown the average time doctors spend with patients one-on-one has been reduced significantly in managed care environments (1). The public had been fed drive-through fast-food for decades, but it was not about to quietly tolerate being fed *fast-food* style medicine.

The old models of medicine are breaking down in many important ways. This break down is happening particularly with the chronic degenerative disorders of our time: diabetes, high blood pressure, arthritis, chronic fatigue, and fibromyalgia, to name a few. The public is no longer satisfied with the limited answers and therapeutic options they have been receiving in regards to cancer, heart disease, and other common, lethal diseases. It cannot be denied that high-tech medicine excels in crisis situations, such as traumatic injuries, acute infectious disease, and critical care. However, despite the staggering amount of money being spent on crisis-centered medicine, after factors such as improved infant mortality and the control of infectious disease by modern public health measures and antibiotics are considered, the average life-span of a human being has not been increased nearly to the predicted levels that were postulated several decades ago, nor has the quality of life in the elderly been significantly improved. This is particularly true for lower socioeconomic segments of the population (2). Sure, we all hear about life expectancy statistically going up by several months every few years. However, the big leaps in life expectancy really occurred in the first half of the twentieth century due to better public health and the development of antibiotic medications to treat serious acute bacterial infections. The gains made have been relatively small over the past several decades and are much less than we had been promised would occur with modern advanced medicine. The small amount of increased life expectancy that has been gained does not seem enough given the massive expenditures in our healthcare system. Much of the healthcare money is being spent to gain a few months of life in elderly people who generally have a poor quality of life due to disabilities and maladies caused by growing old. Many health advocates now suggest we not measure our progress mainly by the extension of lifespan (increasing age of mortality) for a very unhealthy population by small amounts but by reducing the level of disability (compression of morbidity) while we are alive. Healthcare now accounts for $1 out of every $6, or $2 trillion, spent in the U.S. economy. It is expected to account for $1 of every $5, or $4 trillion, in another decade as announced in early 2007 by economists at the Centers for Medicare and Medicaid Services. This means a rise in out-of-pocket expenditures per person, such as the co-pays for medicine and office visits, from about $850 per year in 2007 to about $1,400 by 2016, a 5.3 percent annual increase (3). Are we getting our money's worth?

More and more patients go to their doctors with many vague complaints that seem to overlap each other. These complaints are often not bad enough to warrant a specific medical diagnosis. A typical modern patient does not fit the crisis-centered medical model developed in the early part of the twentieth century when medicine focused on solving acute situations such as deadly bacterial and viral outbreaks. Today's complicated patient is often shuffled from one specialist to another without receiving viable answers to her health concerns. Instead, the patient is often put on multiple drugs to suppress her multiple symptoms. Eventually, if she returns to her doctor enough times, she may even be diagnosed with an apparent *Prozac deficiency*. The patient begins to feel that her physical complaints are all in her head since the doctor cannot figure it out and she was given a medication for depression. This is not only arrogant and lazy medicine; it's just plain bad medicine. Although, consider the dilemma of the average doctor in the modern managed-care environment. What else can he or she do in five minutes? Get to know you? Know your diet and lifestyle? Know your life stressors? Not likely.

People have begun to realize that they have to take control of and assume the responsibility for their own health. To retain their vitality and achieve a greater level of wellness, many people are trying to learn all that they can about alternative health methods, only to be confronted with the previously alluded to plethora of contradictory information.

4

In this short to-the-point book, I used my experience as a university professor of alternative and integrative medicine and my experience as an alternative medicine practitioner who practices within a multi-specialty integrative medicine clinic to give you some insight into the alternative medicine revolution. You will find common sense information on diet, vitamins, herbs, and more. To help you in your quest for wellness, I have also outlined major alternative healthcare providers available to you. Included are my opinions on the strengths and weaknesses of each type of therapy and practitioner's approach. While this may be somewhat politically incorrect, and knowing not all my colleagues will be very happy with me, I feel the reader deserves this information. After all, this is not a particularly politically correct subject to begin with. Let us begin the journey through the often confusing but fascinating world of alternative medicine. Let me teach you how to make rational choices and construct an individualized wellness program unique to your needs.

References:

1. Hu, P. and D.B. Reuben, Effects of managed care on the length of time that elderly patients spend with physicians during ambulatory visits: National Ambulatory Medical Care Survey. Med Care, 2002. 40(7): p. 606-13.

2. Singh, G.K. and M. Siahpush, Widening socioeconomic inequalities in US life expectancy, 1980-2000. Int J Epidemiol, 2006. 35(4): p. 969-79.

3. Freking K. Health care may be 1/5 of what you spend. Associated Press. February 21, 2007.

Diet

Of all of the subjects discussed in this book, none is more important, more emotional, or more confusing than diet. The way people eat is very personal. It is driven by many things; including emotions, peer pressure, and socialization. People's dietary habits are often set in stone and extremely hard to change without a very strong, personal commitment. However, there is probably nothing that has a greater affect on your overall health and longevity than your diet. No amount of vitamin supplements, exercise, or stress management can change that fact. Oh sure, they can all help, but a good healthy diet is the foundation of a healthy lifestyle.

Let's say you realize your diet is not the greatest and you are ready to try and make a positive change. What do you do first? Go to the bookstore? Your confusion would be just beginning. I'm sure you have seen the many diet books out there: *The New Pritikin Program, Eat More, Weigh Less* by Ornish, *The McDougall Program, Dr. Atkin's New Diet Revolution, The Zone* by Sears, *The South Beach Diet* by Agatston, *Eat Right 4 Your Type* by D'Adamo, and *The Paleo Diet* by Cordain just to name a few (1-7). Many of the diets plainly contradict one another. Which one do you believe? Which one is right? Well in a way, they all may be right. You see, no diet is right for every person. We are all individuals with different bodies, biochemical idiosyncrasies, and preferences. Scientists and physicians call this *genetic polymorphism*, but they rarely pay any attention to it when recommending diets and doling out health advice. The government certainly does not consider individuality when making public dietary guidelines. It is easier to try and fit everyone into one big box. In fact, all of the above mentioned diets have their place and have worked wonders for particular individuals. In my clinical practice, I have seen positive benefits from all of these diets. The trick is to figure out which style of dietary consumption agrees with you and is rational in your specific situation. It may require a bit of trial and error. However, the effort will be well worth it if you can avoid or correct things like obesity, diabetes, and heart disease, or if you just want to feel more energetic and have greater vitality.

During the past several decades the trend in dietary guidelines has been to emphasize the restriction of saturated animal fats and advocate the liberal consumption of complex carbohydrates such as breads, cereals, and grains. There are several reasons for this:

One reason is that a major study called the *Framingham Study* produced its first publications in the early seventies and has resulted in numerous publications since that time. The study established a potential link between saturated animal fats, high cholesterol levels, and heart disease (8). In anticipation of the release of this information, the food industry mounted an unprecedented campaign to get the American public to consume hydrogenated oil products, such as margarine, instead of butter which contains animal fat. It is more profitable to bubble hydrogen gas through inexpensive vegetable oil, add some yellow dye, salt, and often a heavy metal catalyst, to make margarine that can be sold for a much higher profit than the animal-derived butter. Unfortunately for the public, during the process of hydrogenation (making oils semi-solid at room temperature), some fat molecules are reconfigured into fats called *trans-fats*. *Trans-fats* cause a multitude of problems within the body. In fact, data suggests these *trans-fats* may cause more heart disease than saturated animal fats (9-12). This issue is now receiving some traction in public discourse; recently several municipalities, including New York City, have begun to limit or ban the use of trans-fat-containing oils in restaurants and fast-food establishments. While it does add somewhat to production costs, European countries have moved to strictly regulate the amount of *trans-fats* in all products containing hydrogenated oil (13). The United States on the other hand has not done so to date. Is this possibly due to pressure from the politically powerful and financially strong food industry?

Secondly, during this same time period high carbohydrate diets were being touted by endurance athletes. Many athletes and sports trainers felt better performance was achieved when a high carbohydrate diet is consumed. This is called *"carbohydrate loading."* The benefits of this type of diet on athletic performance were automatically applied to the average person by many nutritionists. While this dietary strategy may make physiological sense for the high demand, endurance athlete, does it make sense for the rather sedentary, average American?

Thirdly, studies using diets such as those advocated by cardiologists like Drs. Pritikin, Ornish, and MacDougall were showing that the incidence of elevated cholesterol and heart disease, as well as diabetes, can be lowered by following a greatly reduced fat diet with liberal amounts of complex carbohydrates (14-15). Unfortunately, the average person often finds these diets to be boring, non-palatable, and extremely hard to stick to. It is commonly described as *"eating like a rabbit."* It has been suggested by many that it is actually the very high fiber component of the diets in these studies that have the major therapeutic effect rather than the low-fat / high-carbohydrate profile. The average person has a difficult time eating the prescribed amount of fiber required by these diets. If strictly adhered to these diets seem to work, but are these diets the only way? Are they right for all individuals?

As far back as the 1970's, authors began to challenge the belief that low fat / high complex carbohydrate diets were the only way to lose weight and control diseases such as diabetes and heart disease. In fact, the late Dr. Robert Atkins in his book *The New Diet Revolution* contended that it is the high carbohydrate content in the standard American diet that actually induces diabetes and leads to obesity, high cholesterol, and heart disease. Other books then jumped on this bandwagon, such as the *Carbohydrate Addict's Diet* by Heller and Heller, *Sugar Busters* by Leighton-Steward and Bethea, and *Protein Power* by Eades and Eades (16-18). According to the theory proposed in these books, excess carbohydrates the body is forced to convert to fat are actually what leads to high blood fats and obesity. However, it is much easier for the public to conceptualize that *fat makes you fat,* rather than to understand the biochemistry involved in the concept of *sugar being converted to fat and making you fat.* Just look at all the overweight people who liberally eat so called *no fat* or *low fat* foods without any consideration for the staggering amount of "junk" carbohydrates they contain. After all, what are cattle fed to quickly plump them up for slaughter? That's right.....corn, mainly a carbohydrate, not a fat. The fact of the matter is either fat or sugar can make you fat if they are over-consumed. It is true, though, that most people in the United States probably eat too many carbohydrates, and those eaten are for the most part the wrong kind such as simple sugars from sodas, fruity drinks, candy, and baked goods. While these may be the most obvious of the troublesome carbohydrates there certainly are others. You may have been told that eating lots of breads, pastas, potatoes, or rice is good for you. In fact, many people become carbohydrate *junkies.* If they do not eat bread, pasta, potatoes, or rice in large amounts at every meal, they simply do not feel satisfied. Luckily, this addictive-like effect does diminish after several days when less of these foods are consumed. These people often find it difficult, if not impossible, to lose weight by simply reducing their calorie consumption and eating *low fat.* Already obese, dieting further often reduces their metabolism resulting in a plateau effect with little or no weight loss. When dieting is stopped, they may experience an even greater weight gain when they inevitably resume their normal bad ways of eating.

The Atkins, or *ketogenic,* diet may seem like a radical solution, but it often does work, at least temporarily, if done in a controlled way. The diet strictly limits carbohydrates of any kind but allows you to liberally eat protein and fat-based foods. While this may sound extremely appealing to some, it can become too rich a diet to tolerate over long periods of time and often results in significant constipation. On the other hand, patients do not feel as hungry or deprived as they do on severely restricted caloric and low-fat diets. With very few carbohydrates coming in, the body is forced to break down fat in order to create energy. This results in the body depleting its fat reserves, and a significant weight loss usually takes place in a fairly brief amount of time. Unfortunately, it also results in a build-up of ketones, the metabolic waste product of fats. This explains the formal name of this dietary approach, which is the "ketogenic diet". The purpose of this diet is to cause the formation of ketones. The formation of ketones means you are burning fat. The amount of ketones produced by this diet must be tightly controlled since excess ketones can cause your body to become acidic. If ketones reach a dangerous level, a person can become comatose. This is why Dr. Atkins suggests using "Ketostix", available at any drug store, in order to easily monitor your urine and assure that ketones are being kept at safe levels.

Unfortunately, many people start this type of low-carbohydrate diet on the advice of friends or they buy Dr. Atkins' book but read only the book's front and back covers and proceed to put themselves into unmonitored ketosis. Often times, they don't read enough of the book to get to the part about re-introducing carbohydrates back into your diet as you approach your target weight in order to find your "carbohydrate threshold". This is the point at which you are no longer in ketosis and are also not consuming excess carbohydrates. This point is different for each person. It is unique and individualized to you and can only be found by reintroducing carbohydrates back into your diet and monitoring your urine making sure it is barely free of ketones. This is the "maintenance" phase of the diet Atkins proposes, but many people never learn about it.

While the ketogenic diet is probably not a great long-term diet, and many have criticized it for allowing large amounts of fatty and low-fiber foods, I have seen it facilitate significant weight loss and at least a temporary improvement in cholesterol and lipid levels in individuals who were resistant to just about every other method (15). The health benefits of reducing obesity in these people cannot be overstated and must be weighed against the potential risk of consuming additional animal fats. Is this diet right for everyone? Once again, probably not, but if you are significantly overweight and have not had luck with other approaches, it is worth a trying. I recommend it be done under the supervision of a doctor or nutritionist with experience in this approach.

The approach advocated by Barry Sears, Ph.D. in his book, *Entering the Zone*, may be a bit more palatable to dieters and critics alike. Its approach is not as radical as the Atkins diet and is a much easier and healthier diet for the long-term in my opinion. The maintenance phase of *The South Beach Diet* also adopts this moderate strategy. This approach also promotes the theory that most people eat too many carbohydrates, which can imbalance blood sugar, destabilize insulin levels, and lead to chronic inflammation. Of course, all of this can result in obesity, diabetes, heart disease, and other problems. Dr. Sears suggests that an acceptable hormonal balance can be achieved if the diet is made up of approximately 40% calories from carbohydrates, 30% from protein, and 30% from fat. However, unlike Atkins, Sears strongly stipulates the carbohydrates should be complex and non-starchy (simple sugars, potatoes, pasta, and bread are de-emphasized), the protein should be lean (fish and poultry are encouraged), and the fat should be of the monounsaturated variety whenever possible (olive oil, nuts, seeds, etc.). (See *Table I* for the carbohydrate content of many common foods). This dietary balance differs significantly from the 70% carbohydrate, 15% protein, 15% fat diet long advocated by conventional dieticians and the American Dietetic Association. As Sears points out, whether it is the failure of the high carbohydrate / low-fat diet or the inability of the public to adhere to it, the promotion of this dietary approach to the American public for the past thirty years has resulted in a population with more and more obesity, diabetes, high blood pressure, and heart disease. The thirty year experiment is a failure and should be discontinued as a *one-size-fits-all* approach to food consumption. There has finally been some realization of this and some, but not enough, changes in public policy have emerged as can be seen in the new revised government food pyramid and dietary guidelines (www.mypyramid.gov). The pyramid does not provide enough understandable and practical information for most people to incorporate it into their daily lives (19-20).

Table I: Carbohydrate Content of Foods

3 percent	6 percent	15 percent	20 percent	25 percent or greater
UNLIMITED AMOUNTS	REASONABLE PORTION	USE IN MODERATION	AVOID	AVOID
Asparagus	Beans, string	Artichokes	Barley	Artichoke pasta
Bamboo shoots	Carrots, raw	Artichokes, Jerusalem	Beans, dried	Baked goods
Bean Sprouts	Eggplant	Beans, Kidney	Beans, lima	Breads
Beet greens	Kohlrabi	Beans, soy	Buckwheat	Candies
Broccoli	Leeks	Beets	Bulgur	Cookies
Brussel sprouts	Okra	Hominy	Millet	Corn flour, chips, etc.
Cabbage	Olives	Miso	Oats	Corn, sweet
Cauliflower	Onions	Parsnips	Other grains	Crackers
Celery	Peppers, green or red	Peas, green	Other legumes (beans)	Pasta (macaroni)- any type
Chard, Swiss	Pimento	Pumpkin	Quinoa	Pastries
Chicory	Rutabagas	Squash, winter	Rye	Pies
Chives	Tomato juice	Tofu	Wild rice	Potato, sweet
Collards	Tomatoes	Tomato paste		Potato, white
Cucumber	Turnips	Tomato sauce	Apples	Rice, brown
Dandelion greens			Blueberries	Sugar
Endive	Avocado	Apricots	Cherries	Wheat and wheat flour
Kale	Cantaloupe	Blackberries	Grapes	Yams
Lettuce	Cranberries	Gooseberries	Kumquats	Yucca root
Mushrooms	Grapefruit	Guava	Loganberries	
Mustard greens	Lemons	Papaya	Mango	Bananas
Parsley	Limes	Peaches	Mulberries	Dates
Radishes	Melon, any type	Plums	Pears	Figs
Spinach	Oranges	Raspberries	Pineapple	Fruit juices
Squash, summer	Rhubarb		Pomegranate	Other dried fruits
Watercress	Strawberries			Prunes
Zucchini	Tangerines			Raisins
	Watermelon			

Courtesy of: Robban Sica, M.D. (Orange, CT)

15

The Zone dietary strategy also has the advantage of being easy to follow. When making food selections, it is important to try and limit breads, potatoes, pastas, and even rice to complimentary proportions, rather than as a major element of the meal. The carbohydrates you choose should come more from non-starchy vegetables such as broccoli, squash, cauliflower, greens, etc., than from potatoes, pasta, rice, and bread. These colorful vegetables also contain large amounts of vitamins and minerals, as well as substantial amounts of antioxidant and anti-carcinogenic phytonutrients (substances in vegetables and fruits which reduce oxidative stress and cancer). High-sugar containing vegetables, such as carrots and corn, should be avoided or occasionally consumed in small amounts. Dr. Sears suggests imagining your plate cut into thirds, with 2/3 consisting of a non-starchy vegetable source that has been steamed or sautéed in a little olive oil, and the other 1/3 consisting of a lean protein, such as chicken, turkey, fish, tofu, beans, etc., that has been cooked in a healthy way (broiling, baking, or sautéing in olive oil). This is much easier than weighing foods or counting points as is required by some dietary plans. It will usually give you the desired 40/30/30 micronutrient ratio, or close to it, while at the same time provide you with the required vitamins, minerals, and phytonutrients needed in a healthy diet. However, selection of quality carbohydrates, proteins, and fats is critical!

When suggesting this style of eating to selected patients of mine, I have received some interesting reactions and comments. One of my favorites is: *I can't eat like that. I'm Italian!* I then go on to explain to the person that if they were to travel throughout Italy they would find that meal generally consists of just what I described: a main dish that includes a healthy vegetable and a lean protein (often chicken, veal, or fish), with possibly a little pasta on the side, and a green salad. The pasta is rarely served in the quantities Americans are used to eating. It is seldom the *bed* for which the entire meal is laid upon, as it is in American-Italian cooking. Indeed, most Mediterranean cultures eat in this healthy fashion. Nutritionists have discussed this for many years and refer to it as the *French or Mediterranean paradox*. Why do these cultures eat more fat than is advocated by American dieticians, and yet they still have lower incidences of obesity, diabetes, and heart disease (21-22)? In fact, the Greek island of Crete's population consumes a very high fat diet and has 40% less heart disease than Americans. Of course, there are many factors that play a role in this phenomenon. You need to take into account the fact that the foods consumed by these cultures are mostly fresh and non-processed, they ingest a moderate portion of antioxidant-rich and blood thinning red wine with most meals, and walk as part of their daily routine. Nevertheless, these facts certainly seem to undermine the notion that the low-fat / high-complex carbohydrate diet is the only way to eat and achieve good health. Is this the way everyone should eat? Probably not, but it is something to consider if other dietary styles have not produced results you desire.

Finally, in the book *Paleo Diet* by Loren Cordain the philosophy of the Paleolithic diet is explained and a dietary strategy similar to our distant ancestors is advocated. During the Paleolithic period, which lasted from about 200,000 years ago until about 12,000 years ago, humans mainly lived a hunter-gatherer lifestyle and consumed almost exclusively lean wild meats, fish, vegetables, and fruits. By necessity, these people lived a very active lifestyle which involved far more exercise than humans presently are accustomed to. Over this vast amount of time, the human genome (our genetic code) became very compatible with this style of eating and activity level. This theory suggests that since this period lasted for so long humans slowly became accustomed to this diet and lifestyle, while those individuals who were not compatible with it were naturally eliminated from the gene pool.

Starting about 12,000 years ago in the Middle East and about 6,000 years ago in Scandinavia and the British Isles new foods, including farmed grains, milk, and meat from domesticated animals began to be introduced due to rapidly increasing human populations and the advent of more modern farming techniques. Advocates of the Paleolithic dietary approach claim that this rapid introduction of new foods over a comparatively short period of time created problems for humans. These include genetic incompatibility and intolerance to many of these new foods, which may correlate with the rise in many of our current degenerative diseases, such as heart disease, stroke, some cancers (i.e. prostate, breast, colon), many autoimmune diseases and a variety of chronic degenerative diseases (i.e. Parkinson's, Alzheimer's) to name a few. Interestingly enough, new research into autoimmune diseases (where the body attacks its own tissues) has been linked to immune intolerance to food and microbial proteins. For example, those individuals who do not tolerate gluten in certain grains like wheat, barley and rye, may be diagnosed with Celiac disease (an inflammatory disorder of the small intestine) and also have a much higher prevalence of autoimmune diseases of the thyroid such as Grave's and Hashimoto's disease (23-24). This process is known as *molecular mimicry* and involves the immune system reacting to a protein from the food we consume or a bacteria which we are infected by, but also then cross-reacting to a structurally similar protein which is part of a tissue in our body (25-26). In other words, the immune system becomes confused between the two proteins, one "foreign" and one "self". There has also emerged in the scientific literature a molecular mimicry connection between allergy to cow's milk proteins and/or cow's milk insulin and the development of Type I diabetes, an autoimmune disease against receptor proteins of the pancreas (27-29). In fact, many of these newly introduced foods after the Paleolithic period seem to be those implicated in triggering the auto-immune and inflammatory reactions which are at the heart of many modern chronic diseases.

A diet of lean meat, fish, fruits and vegetables is now considered to represent a Paleolithic diet and such a diet is that to which humans may be most genetically adapted (30-31). In a Paleolithic diet, protein makes up about 25-30% of the calories and is derived almost exclusively from lean meats (preferably organic free-range or grass fed) and fish. This contrasts with the Standard American Diet (S.A.D.) that consists usually of only 10-15% protein derived from high fat meats, grains, dairy products, and legumes. Paleolithic carbohydrates made up about 30-35% of the calorie intake and were gained mainly from fruits and vegetables having a low glycemic index (did not raise blood sugar or insulin very much) and were also abundant in micro-nutrients (vitamins and minerals) and fiber. By contrast, the S.A.D. contains 50-60% of calories, nearly twice that of the Paleolithic diet, from carbohydrates mainly derived from grains and refined sugars with fruits and vegetables being a minor supply. Paleolithic diets contained about 35-40% of calories from fats but consisted mainly of monosaturated and polyunsaturated fats, which included substantial amounts of beneficial omega-3-fatty acids from fish and other sources. The main fat sources were lean wild animals, fish, and nuts, as opposed to the S.A.D. that contains mainly saturated fat from red meats and dairy products, as well as trans-fatty acids from margarines and processed baked goods. The Paleolithic diet also contained approximately three times more micronutrients (vitamins, minerals, antioxidants) than does the S.A.D. The Paleolithic dietary make-up is remarkably similar in most ways to the *Zone* approach I discussed earlier, although it would be more restrictive of grains and legumes. This Paleolithic approach is one I have found works very well with my patients and one which I am becoming more and more comfortable with as more data emerges on autoimmune and chronic inflammatory diseases.

Please consult *Table 1* to determine the approximate carbohydrate content of many common foods in order to help you select foods which are not too high in simple sugars and starches.

General Dietary Guidelines:

If any of the descriptions of the different diets reviewed in this chapter seem to resonate with you, I would encourage you to consider consulting one of the books specific to that approach for a more detailed explanation (See the *Recommended Reading* section in the *Resource* chapter of the book). Remember, no particular strategy of food consumption is perfect for every person so you may have to experiment a little to see what seems to work for you as an individual. However, there are some general suggestions I would like to make that can actually be applied to any dietary style:

1.   *Eat fresh, non-processed foods whenever possible.* One of my mentors once said to me, *The less doctored the foods that you eat are, the less doctoring you will need.* I believe this to be truer today than ever before. Pre-packaged convenience foods are obviously full of additives, preservatives, and all sorts of unnatural chemicals you probably cannot pronounce. Go ahead, read an ingredients label on a packaged food product. I dare you! After all, it is just plain old common sense to try to avoid chemically-laden *science* foods whenever possible. Keep this in mind while shopping: Stay around the outside edges of most grocery stores. That is where the *real* food is! Have you ever noticed foods such as fresh produce, meats, and dairy are found around the outside perimeter of the store while all the *junk* and *science* foods are in the middle aisles? This is for a reason. Since fresh foods have short shelf lives, it is necessary they be sold quickly. Placing them on the periphery allows them to be easily stocked or removed. Enter the middle region at your own peril! The foods there are generally "science-foods" and have very long shelf lives, often because they are full of preservatives and other chemicals. Realistically, there

are times when you must enter this area. Just don't spend much time there.

While it is preferable to buy fresh produce whenever possible, it is important to realize these foods also have their own potential problems. They are often full of pesticide residues and molds that can be harmful when consumed. Wash all fresh vegetables and fruit as completely as possible. Using a veggie-fruit soak and wash is much better at removing the chemicals than using water alone. The potential health concerns of genetically modified produce have yet to be fully understood. However, the benefits of fresh produce still far outweigh concerns associated with them when compared to processed, pre-packaged foods. While there is not a standardized definition of the term *"organic"*, purchasing fresh, organic produce is advisable if it is available in your area and within your budget. Buying organic may lower your exposure to pesticide toxins and genetically altered products. I also tell my patients to apply a simple test to the meal they are about to eat. I tell them to look down at their plate and ask themselves one question: *Could I have purchased this food in the form I purchased it one hundred years ago?* If you ask yourself that question and the answer is yes, then you probably bought fresh food and are well on your way to a healthier diet.

2. *Eat lots of fresh vegetables and reasonable amounts of fruit every day.* The science is very compelling in suggesting that liberal consumption of vegetables

and fruits can help reduce cancer, heart disease, and many other health disorders. It is these fresh whole foods that contain many protective antioxidant and anti-carcinogenic vitamins, minerals, phytonutrients, and fiber. It is important, however, to remember fruits are very high in sugar and can cause difficulty for people with blood sugar control problems. The consumption of fruits, especially dried, also has to be limited to some degree if you are trying to follow one of the previously mentioned higher-protein / lower-carbohydrate diets. Remember the vegetables you select should be fresh, non-processed, and be limited in the sugars and starches if you are trying to consume a moderate carbohydrate diet.

3. ***Limit your consumption of saturated animal fats and hydrogenated trans-fatty acids.*** The excessive, and I stress excessive, consumption of animal fats from meats, eggs (yolks), and dairy has been linked in some studies to the development of cancer and heart disease (32). This does not mean that you should never consume these products, but if you do, you should eat them in moderation and always make the wisest selection possible. For example, try to eat poultry instead of beef or pork the majority of the time, or even better yet, eat the fish. Of particular concern are commercially-raised meats. These animals, including cows, are fed corn and grains rather than their natural diet of grass. Part of the corn, the oil, is converted in their systems to a very inflammatory fat called arachadonic acid. When

we consume the animal's flesh, arachadonic acid is incorporated into our cells. This fat causes our bodies to become much more prone to pain and swelling when our tissues are stressed or traumatized. This may at least partially explain why Western industrialized countries, where most commercially-fed animals are produced and eaten, have such a high incidence of inflammatory disorders like heart disease, pre-diabetes, rheumatoid arthritis, lupus, multiple sclerosis, and other auto-immune related diseases. Free-range grass-fed animals, such as buffalo, do not have this problem, and therefore, are much healthier to consume. Free-range beef and poultry are also available in more areas now, and although more expensive, it is probably worth the investment. After all, some of the healthiest cultures on the planet have traditionally eaten a great deal of animal fat and protein. However, the animals they consume are not commercially raised on grain but are animals that naturally mature consuming foods, like grasses, they were designed to eat.

Unfortunately, many products developed by the food industry to replace animal fats are just as bad or potentially worse. Hydrogenated oils, including margarine, contain *trans-fats* and have been linked to many metabolic problems discussed earlier in this chapter. The flood of new *non-fat* and *low-fat* food products into the marketplace today are not healthy replacement choices, since these are the ultimate *science* foods. They contain a multitude of synthetic chemicals, can result in deficiencies of essential fats and fat soluble vitamins, and can cause many gastrointestinal side effects. The general rule is if you are going to consume products in either of these categories, choose the *natural* fat vs. the *synthetic* fat. *That's right. I'm telling you to use butter instead of margarine!* But use it in moderation!

4.   ***Eat lean protein with every meal.*** It is very important that lean protein is eaten with every meal and snack. Consumption of foods that are high in carbohydrates without balancing them with protein foods can result in lack of energy an hour or two after eating and can result in weight-gain. Protein should always be consumed at breakfast to get a great start to your day. Moderate consumption of eggs (or egg whites) in the morning is suggested. The commercial raising of chickens for modern egg production results in egg yolks with more inflammatory fats, such as arachadonic acid, and less beneficial fats and nutrients due to the feeds given these animals. Free-range, organic eggs are strongly encouraged. Eating the typical bagel, English muffin, or toast alone is not recommended. The use of quality protein powders, such as whey protein (unless you are allergic to dairy), is also a convenient way to consume protein in the morning as well as at other times during the day.

5.   ***Do not over-eat.*** Overeating puts strain on the body in many ways. The actual burning of food to create energy requires many vitamins and minerals. This means if the food that is eaten is not quality fresh food containing large

amount of these vitamins and minerals, the body will use up its storage reserves of these critical nutrients in order to process the excess calories that have been consumed. Many people who overeat are doing so by consuming processed junk foods that do not contain enough of the required vitamins and minerals, such as B-vitamins and magnesium, to adequately metabolize the food itself. The result is a depletion of vitamin and mineral stores which can lead to fatigue and a multitude of health problems.

Many of the break-down products of foods can be somewhat toxic. These substances need to be processed and detoxified by the body. The detoxification of these substances also requires many of the same vitamins and minerals needed to burn the food to produce energy. Therefore, the added need to detoxify substances created by overeating can deplete vitamin and mineral stores in this way as well. This excessive toxic load can also put strain on the liver and kidneys if overeating continues over time.

Consuming more calories than you need over long periods of time eventually leads to obesity. One of the primary risk factors for the most common life-shortening diseases today (diabetes, high blood pressure, heart disease, etc.) is obesity. Study after study has shown the easiest way to extend life-span in animals is to restrict their caloric intake (33). Not enough to starve them, but enough so that they are not consuming excess calories. This is also true for humans.

The American population is overweight and out of shape as a whole. This trend needs to be reversed if we are to truly have a healthy society. One of the first places to start is to discourage overeating. Eat only until your hunger has ceased. It is not necessary to eat until you feel engorged and "stuffed" at every meal. It is just not healthy. Save that feeling for Thanksgiving. Otherwise, eat less and live better and longer!

6. ***Time your eating properly.*** Another important factor in how we eat is the timing in which we consume our meals. The standard American three large meals per day is probably not the best way to maintain stable blood sugar and insulin levels. After all, do you think that Paleolithic man living a hunter-gatherer lifestyle had the luxury of planning three tightly scheduled meals per day? Obviously not, as they likely ate mainly as they found food. This has prompted many nutritionists and physicians to suggest it may be better to eat smaller, more frequent, meals that contain some protein whenever carbohydrates are consumed. While there is a lack of firm scientific data to prove the above hypothesis, and a person with good blood sugar control should be able to tolerate not eating for a considerable amount of time without feeling faint or lethargic, more and more evidence is being collected suggesting that our eating patterns affect our normal hormonal biorhythms. For instance, the studies of researchers such as Fernstrom and Wurtmen into circadian rhythms and amino acid metabolism are supporting the morning intake of protein

(34-35). Clinical trials are now showing that about 50% of individuals subjectively report feeling better when they eat protein-based foods in the morning and consume most of their carbohydrate foods in the evening. This happens to be exactly the opposite of the high carbohydrate breakfast (bagels, cereals, fruit, etc.) and higher protein dinners (meat) of the Standard American Diet (S.A.D.). By the way, isn't that an appropriate acronym for the American diet? The *SAD* diet, which it most certainly is. Furthermore, the coffee consumed with many people's breakfast contains caffeine that also has a profound affect at altering biorhythms and seems to be neutral to these rhythms only between about 3 p.m. and 5 p.m. Oddly enough, this is the British tea time. On further thought, maybe this is not so odd, since many long-time cultural traditions related to diet have some method to their madness or some basis in fact regarding human physiology. For more information on this exciting new area of research on eating to reinforce healthy biorhythms read *The Circadian Prescription* by Dr. Sidney Baker (36).

7. ***Maintain proper fluid consumption.*** We are made up mostly of water. It is the solvent within which the majority of our biochemistry takes place. It is therefore critical that we consume adequate amounts of pure water every day. About six 8-ounce glasses per day is generally recommended, although there is no real hard science to back up this commonly given suggestion. However, it does seem to work. Remember though

this does not include the water in ice cubes in a scotch on the rocks, or the water in coffee, soda, and other fruity drinks. Preferably, it should be plain pure water. Spring water from a trusted source or reverse osmosis filtered water is strongly preferred over tap water. The state of tap water is not as good as government sources would have you believe and is a significant source of chemicals like fluorine, chlorine, and other toxic residues that find their way into the water supply (37). Also, large amounts of water or other liquids should not be consumed with meals since this dilutes the acids in your stomach and may cause digestive difficulties. If you need to drink with meals, drink pure water with the juice of a fresh lemon wedge or two squeezed into it in order to acidify the water. In general, drinking soda and fruity drinks should be eliminated or severely limited. These drinks contain large amounts of sugars and phosphates, and virtually no vitamins or synergistic nutrients to metabolize the large amount of sugar in them. Unfortunately, these drinks are the beverages of choice for our population, particularly our children. A nice alternative to soda is to fill a glass with ice, add about 2/3 sparkling water, and 1/3 fresh fruit juice. The result is a healthy and refreshing fruit spritzer that is a far better choice than soda or sugar-laden fruit drinks.

8.   *Limit alcohol consumption*. There has been a great deal of contradictory information regarding the consumption of alcohol over the past several years. Some studies and authorities claim alcohol should not be consumed in any

quantity, while others claim that a moderate amount of alcohol may be beneficial (38-39). It is established that consuming significant amounts of alcohol is not healthy and can lead to health problems. Chronic excessive alcohol consumption can put stress on the liver and eventually may lead to degeneration and cirrhosis of the liver. Even moderate amounts of alcohol on a daily basis (3-4 drinks per day) can lead to elevated blood liver enzymes in some individuals, which are indicators of liver destruction. Alcohol is also very dehydrating and hard on the lining of the intestines, potentially leading to ulcers or a "leaky gut." A leaky gut is essentially where the intestinal lining degrades and lets more substances through from the foods you eat into the blood stream than is normal. This can ultimately result in a plethora of food allergies and added toxicity for body. If one abuses alcohol to the point of becoming an alcoholic, a large array of health problems can ensue including ruptures of the esophagus, neurological degeneration, and liver failure.

On the other hand, many cultures have traditionally consumed a small amount of alcohol with meals and don't seem to suffer adverse effects from it. It appears they may actually derive some benefit from the alcohol. The Mediterranean cultures, such as the Italians, French, and Greeks, usually consume wine with meals. However, their daily alcohol consumption is not generally excessive and often in the form of red wine. Red wine contains many antioxidants, like resveratrol and pterostilbene, from the purple grapes used in wine making. These antioxidants have beneficial effects on the body (40-42). Alcohol also serves to thin the blood slightly which can result in blood that is somewhat less sticky, and therefore, less likely to stick to the walls of arteries and form clots. This is similar to the effect of taking a baby aspirin each day in order to thin the blood. Many people with a history of stroke and heart attack take baby aspirin daily under the advice of their physician. Alcohol can also help lower the "bad" cholesterol (LDL), while increasing the "good" cholesterol (HDL) (43-44). These phenomena probably account for the lower incidence of heart attacks and stroke in those who drink moderately. Alcohol has also been shown to lower blood pressure and the incidence of respiratory diseases, some cancers, and a host of other health conditions. Many studies are confirming that moderate alcohol consumption (no more than 2-3 drinks per day) can actually lead to better overall health. A recent study conducted at Harvard revealed a 21-28% decrease in death rates from all causes in men who were moderate drinkers versus abstainers. A similar study in China showed a 20% reduction. The National Institute on Alcohol Abuse and Alcoholism reported moderate intake of alcohol lengthened life span by 3% among white male drinkers when compared to non-drinkers, while The Harvard Nurses Health Study of over 85,000 female subjects clearly showed that those who drank a moderate amount of alcohol on a regular basis had reduced mortality rates.

In summary, the excessive consumption of alcohol can have adverse effects on the liver, gut lining, and other systems of the body and can lead to significant disability and early death. Moderate intake of alcohol may actually afford some health benefits, although this is still a controversial and hotly debated point. I think common sense will tell you that enjoying an alcoholic beverage occasionally is fine. Just do not drink more than two or three drinks when you do decide to drink. If you enjoy wine with your dinner that is also fine. Just make it one or two glasses and select the red wine over the white wine the majority of the time. If you are on blood thinning medications, you should check with your doctor before consuming alcohol. Remember, a little goes a long way. Don't abuse it and you will be fine. The Russian proverb may have said it best: *Drink a glass of schnapps after your soup and steal a ruble from your doctor.* Just remember, it says ONE glass of schnapps!

9. *Supplement your diet with critical vitamins and minerals.* See the next chapter on vitamins and minerals and the chapter on "Creating Your Unique Nutrition Program" for details.

10. Consider taking a *Comprehensive Metabolic Profile* to learn which foods work best with your unique immune response. Learn more about this testing and how you can find a practitioner in your area who can order this test for you by visiting *healthyrevolution.info*

General Dietary Guidelines

1. Eat fresh non-processed foods whenever possible

2. Eat lots of fresh vegetables and reasonable amounts of fruit every day

3. Limit your consumption of saturated animal fats and hydrogenated trans-fatty acids

4. Eat lean protein with every meal or snack

5. Do not over-eat

6. Time your eating properly

7. Maintain proper fluid consumption

8. Avoid or limit alcohol consumption

9. Supplement your diet with critical vitamins and minerals.

10. Take a Comprehensive Metabolic Profile to determine your unique diet and supplement needs by visiting healthyrevolution.info.

References:

1. Pritikin R. New Pritikin Program. New York: Pocket; 1991.

2. Ornish D. Eat More, Weight Less: Dr. Dean Ornish's Life Choice Program for Losing Weight Safetly While Eating Abundantly. New York: Harper Collins; 2000.

3. MacDougall J, MacDougal M. The MacDougal Program for Maximum Weight Loss. New York: Plume; 1995.

4. Atkins R. Dr. Atkin's New Diet Revolution. 3rd ed. New York: M. Evans; 2002.

5. Sears B. Enter the Zone. New York: Regan Books/Harper Collins; 1995.

6. Agaston A. The South Beach Diet. New York: Rodale, Inc.; 2003.

7. Corain L. The Paleo Diet. Hoboken: Wiley Publishing; 2002.

8. Posner, B.M., et al., *Diet and heart disease risk factors in adult American men and women: the Framingham Offspring-Spouse nutrition studies*. Int J Epidemiol, 1993. **22**(6): p. 1014-25.

9. Costa, A.G., J. Bressan, and C.M. Sabarense, *[Trans fatty acids: foods and effects on health]*. Arch Latinoam Nutr, 2006. **56**(1): p. 12-21.

10. Mozaffarian, D., *Trans fatty acids - effects on systemic inflammation and endothelial function*. Atheroscler Suppl, 2006. **7**(2): p. 29-32.

11. Odegaard, A.O. and M.A. Pereira, *Trans fatty acids, insulin resistance, and type 2 diabetes*. Nutr Rev, 2006. **64**(8): p. 364-72.

12. Oh, K., et al., *Dietary fat intake and risk of coronary heart disease in women: 20 years of follow-up of the nurses' health study*. Am J Epidemiol, 2005. **161**(7): p. 672-9.

13. Stender, S. and J. Dyerberg, *Influence of trans fatty acids on health*. Ann Nutr Metab, 2004. **48**(2): p. 61-6.

14. Anderson, J.W. and K. Ward, *High-carbohydrate, high-fiber diets for insulin-treated men with diabetes mellitus.* Am J Clin Nutr, 1979. **32**(11): p. 2312-21.

15. Connor, W.E., P.B. Duell, and S.L. Connor, *Benefits and hazards of dietary carbohydrate.* Curr Atheroscler Rep, 2005. **7**(6): p. 428-34.

16. Eades M, MD E. Protein Power. New York: Bantam Books; 1997.

17. Steward H, Bethea M. The New Sugar Busters. New York: Ballantine Books; 2002.

18. Heller R, Heller R. The Carbohydrate Addicts Diet. New York: Signet Publishers; 1993.

19. Britten, P., J. Haven, and C. Davis, *Consumer Research for Development of Educational Messages for the MyPyramid Food Guidance System.* J Nutr Educ Behav, 2006. **38 Suppl 2**: p. S108-23.

20. Gao, X., et al., *The 2005 USDA Food Guide Pyramid is associated with more adequate nutrient intakes within energy constraints than the 1992 Pyramid.* J Nutr, 2006. **136**(5): p. 1341-6.

21. *Bellisle, F.,* Nutrition and health in France: dissecting a paradox. J Am Diet Assoc, 2005. **105**(12): p. 1870-3.

22. de Lorgeril, M., et al., *Mediterranean diet and the French paradox: two distinct biogeographic concepts for one consolidated scientific theory on the role of nutrition in coronary heart disease.* Cardiovasc Res, 2002. **54**(3): p. 503-15.

23. Akcay, M.N. and G. Akcay, *The presence of the antigliadin antibodies in autoimmune thyroid diseases.* Hepatogastroenterology, 2003. **50 Suppl 2**: p. cclxxix-cclxxx.

24. Fanciulli, G., et al., *Screening for celiac disease in patients with autoimmune thyroid disease: from research studies to daily clinical practice.* Ann Ital Med Int, 2005. **20**(1): p. 39-44.

25. Bach, J.F., *Infections and autoimmune diseases.* J Autoimmun, 2005. **25 Suppl**: p. 74-80.

26. Franceschi, F., et al., *Helicobacter pylori infection in patients with Hashimoto's thyroiditis.* Helicobacter, 2004. **9**(4): p. 369.

27. Lammi, N., M. Karvonen, and J. Tuomilehto, *Do microbes have a causal role in type 1 diabetes?* Med Sci Monit, 2005. **11**(3): p. RA63-9.

28. Strycharz, M., K. Bartecka, and M. Polz-Dacewicz, *The role of viruses in the etiopathogenesis of diabetes mellitus.* Ann Univ Mariae Curie Sklodowska [Med], 2004. **59**(1): p. 257-60.

29. Vaarala, O., *Is type 1 diabetes a disease of the gut immune system triggered by cow's milk insulin?* Adv Exp Med Biol, 2005. **569**: p. 151-6.

30. Mann, N.J., *Paleolithic nutrition: what can we learn from the past?* Asia Pac J Clin Nutr, 2004. **13**(Suppl): p. S17.

31. O'Keefe, J.H., Jr. and L. Cordain, *Cardiovascular disease resulting from a diet and lifestyle at odds with our Paleolithic genome: how to become a 21st-century hunter-gatherer.* Mayo Clin Proc, 2004. **79**(1): p. 101-8.

32. Granados, S., et al., *Dietary lipids and cancer.* Nutr Hosp, 2006. **21 Suppl 2**: p. 42-52, 44-54.

33. Holliday, R., *Aging is no longer an unsolved problem in biology.* Ann N Y Acad Sci, 2006. **1067**: p. 1-9.

34. Fernstrom, J.D. and R.J. Wurtman, *Control of brain serotonin levels by the diet.* Adv Biochem Psychopharmacol, 1974. **11**(0): p. 133-42.

35. Fernstrom, J.D., et al., *Diurnal variations in plasma concentrations of tryptophan, tryosine, and other neutral amino acids: effect of dietary protein intake.* Am J Clin Nutr, 1979. **32**(9): p. 1912-22.

36. MacDonald Baker S, Baar K. The Circadian Prescription. New York: Perigee Trade; 2001.

37. Donohue, J.M. and J.C. Lipscomb, *Health advisory values for drinking water contaminants and the methodology for determining acute exposure values.* Sci Total Environ, 2002. **288**(1-2): p. 43-9.

38. Djousse, L. and J.M. Gaziano, *Alcohol Consumption and Risk of Heart Failure in the Physicians' Health Study I.* Circulation, 2006.

39. Gigleux, I., et al., *Moderate alcohol consumption is more cardioprotective in men with the metabolic syndrome.* J Nutr, 2006. **136**(12): p. 3027-32.

40. Baur, J.A., et al., *Resveratrol improves health and survival of mice on a high-calorie diet.* Nature, 2006. **444**(7117): p. 337-42.

41. Baur, J.A. and D.A. Sinclair, *Therapeutic potential of resveratrol: the in vivo evidence.* Nat Rev Drug Discov, 2006. **5**(6): p. 493-506.

42. Corder, R., et al., *Oenology: red wine procyanidins and vascular health.* Nature, 2006. **444**(7119): p. 566.

43. Mukamal, K.J., S.E. Chiuve, and E.B. Rimm, *Alcohol consumption and risk for coronary heart disease in men with healthy lifestyles.* Arch Intern Med, 2006. **166**(19): p. 2145-50.

44. Schroder, H., et al., *Myocardial infarction and alcohol consumption: A population-based case-control study.* Nutr Metab Cardiovasc Dis, 2006.

Vitamins
(And Other Supplements)

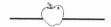

At the beginning of the last chapter on diet, I stated that of all the topics discussed in this book none may be more controversial or confusing than diet. Well, maybe I was forgetting about vitamins and nutritional supplementation. We have all been frustrated by the ever-changing vitamin information reported by the media. It seems that today vitamin C helps prevent colds, while tomorrow it doesn't. Yesterday vitamin E helped prevent heart disease, but today it does not. Why can't the experts get it straight and make up their minds? To understand why this situation exists, you may have to look at the politics behind the question.

Why are vitamins and supplements so controversial, and do I really need them?

For decades conventional Western medicine has seemingly downplayed the importance of vitamins and other supplements. Western medicine has invested its efforts and money, and medical professionals have invested their professional reputations exclusively in the drug model of healthcare. Make no mistake about it; medicine is a very territorial and financially driven business. The vitamin issue is as much a turf, market-share, and money battle as it is anything else. It is often stated by medical authorities that the public does not have to concern themselves with taking supplemental vitamin pills. In fact, you may even hear that vitamins are just a waste of money and anyone advocating their use is a quack or a snake oil salesman. You may often encounter statements such as *Human beings were not designed to have to take vitamin pills.* Basically, what is being implied is that all the vitamins and minerals you could possibly need are contained in the foods you eat as part of a balanced diet, particularly in wealthy Western countries where food is plentiful. This all sounds logical. However, those advocating that kind of position have made a critical assumption. That assumption being that the average person eats a fresh, non-processed varied diet made up of healthy whole foods. Vitamin pills would not be necessary if people hunted and gathered their food in clean environments and ate only foods intended for their digestive systems. It took millions of years for man's digestive system to evolve to the place it is now. However, when people eat mainly chemically-laden, calorie-rich, nutrient-poor, processed foods of convenience as their daily diet, maybe the concept of supplementing their diets with vitamins and minerals is not so radical after all. Was man meant to need vitamin pills? No more so than he was meant to consume Big Macs, Coca-Cola, and margarine! Previously, I mentioned that some of the politics regarding vitamins and other supplements involves a turf battle and financial issues. So you may be asking yourself, *Where do these concepts fit in to this issue?*

The whole concept of having to supplement the population with certain vitamins and minerals in order for them not to have serious problems related to specific nutrient deficiencies came not from standard medical doctors, but from the public health arena. An example of this is adding iodine to table salt in order to prevent thyroid goiters and hypothyroidism. Goiters were not uncommon in the United States, particularly the northern mid-western states, before this measure was taken. In fact, this region of the United States used to be referred to as the *Goiter Belt* for this very reason. The soil in this area is iodine deficient. At the time goiters were a problem in this region most foods that were consumed by the population were locally grown. The decision was made to add iodine to something that was consumed on a regular basis and table salt was selected. Similar decisions have been made to add certain B vitamins to white bread; since refining, bleaching, and processing the wheat used to make white bread depletes the bread of its vitamin and mineral content leaving not much more than calories behind. Although almost thirty nutrients are depleted during wheat processing, the government requires manufacturers to put back only about eight nutrients. With this addition of nutrients, the phrase *enriched white bread* was coined. This phrase incorrectly makes it seem as if you are receiving added nutrition by consuming a food that has been *enriched*.

While public health officials have won a few battles with the addition of certain nutrients to our foods, this only occurs in the most serious and potentially dangerous of situations. More and more scientific data is emerging that suggests nutritional deficiencies are actually becoming rampant in our population as more and more devitalized and processed foods are consumed. In fact, many behavioral difficulties in our children and violent behaviors in adults have been linked to specific nutritional deficiencies (1-3). However, any effort to address these via supplementation is met with fierce criticism by much of the orthodox medical establishment. Why? These problems can't all be caused by *Ritalin* and *Prozac* deficiencies, can they? The fact that these problems exist encourages the sale of those drugs as well as others. It also fits nicely into the drug model of practice that has developed over many years in crisis-centered conventional Western medicine. Why take the time to address the difficult topic of changing a patient's diet when a prescription can be written for a drug that may mask the problem in a matter of minutes? Besides, who has time to talk about diet in the six to ten minutes that many of the managed-care providers allow a doctor to see a patient?

It is only human nature that those in academic medicine have a tendency not to take seriously and ultimately attack ideas that come from outside their ranks. *After all, if it was such a great idea why didn't we think of it?* seems to be the thinking. This tendency goes back to antiquity and we can look to Galileo as a good example. His seemingly radical scientific ideas were rejected by the intellectuals of the time who viewed him as an outsider. Galileo took his ideas right to the people by writing in Italian rather than Latin, as most *true* scientists of the time were expected to. As it turned out in the end Galileo was right. However, during his lifetime, he was not thought of nor was he recognized as the brilliant scientist that we all know he was.

Interestingly enough, since the benefits of vitamins and minerals were rejected for so long by standard medicine it has been only through the efforts of dedicated scientists and physicians willing to buck the system by going directly to the public that this issue has emerged as a perceived threat to orthodox medicine. However, fundamentally it has been the public who has created the demand that vitamins and minerals be investigated further. There is more and more scientific evidence every day suggesting that vitamins and minerals play a large role in wellness and can actually be used therapeutically to effectively and inexpensively treat some diseases (4,5). A study on behalf of Wyeth Consumer Healthcare using Medicare data from individuals greater than 65 years of age indicates that the use of a daily multivitamin over a five year period could prevent 3.9 billion dollars in Medicare payments. With the cost of multivitamins being 2.3 billion dollars, this represents a net savings of 1.6 billion dollars (6). However, in contrast to this in many ways, there continues to be a strong bias in standard medicine against the use of vitamins. Positive studies on vitamins are often picked apart and condemned, if they are given any attention at all, while negative ones are run up the flagpole almost as triumphs. When the media does report positive results, those results are often portrayed as new discoveries. Oftentimes, similar results had been published years before, and nutritionally-minded physicians had already been using the vitamin in question in that manner for decades. In other words, *The vitamin doesn't work until we are ready to say it does and claim credit for the finding.* In the meantime, negative drug studies and drug side effects are generally tolerated and ignored unless an extreme problem emerges. Examples of some of the under-reported and improperly reported affects of vitamins on health can be illustrated by the data on vitamin E and heart disease. Heart disease is the number one killer in our society, and long-standing scientific evidence clearly shows vitamin E can help in the prevention of this disease (7-12). However, just recently we were told of two studies that implied that vitamin E may actually be dangerous and lead to increased deaths (13,14). What these studies actually showed is the long-term use of *synthetic* vitamin E in the form of d-alpha-tocopherol, which does not include the full spectrum of vitamin E types (alpha, beta, gamma and delta), can potentially be problematic. However, the natural mixture of vitamin E, found in food and quality mixed vitamin E supplements has a long established history of safely preventing disease. However, with one improperly or incompletely reported study, many are willing to throw out their vitamin E, even though there are many more positive studies than negative ones. For instance, The Cambridge Heart Antioxidant Study showed that supplementation with 400IU of vitamin E per day reduced the incidence of heart attacks by 77%, while the Nurse's Health Study, an eight year study on over 87,000 nurses, showed that supplementation with 200IU of vitamin E for 2 years or more resulted in a 41% reduction in cardiovascular disease. The Health Professional's Follow-up Study, a study on almost 40,000 men, revealed a 37% reduction in cardiovascular disease in those subjects consuming at least 400IU of vitamin E per day, while the Atherosclerosis Regression Study reported similar findings. If a new pharmaceutical drug produced results such as these in treating the number one killer disease in Western countries, the media attention these findings would command would be staggering. Why are the public and their physicians virtually unaware of this information? Is there not some form of bias at work here? It must be kept in mind that since this kind of bias has gone on for so long, it would be professional suicide for standard doctors in mass to suddenly do an about face and admit that "OK, maybe we were wrong all the while". It would represent a loss of professional clout and credibility. If a profession loses credibility, the loss often translates into a loss of market share and money. In fact, 1997 was the first year office visits to non-conventional healthcare providers outnumbered those to primary care conventional family physicians in the United States (15). Therein lay the turf battle.

As for finances, it is no secret that the big money that drives medicine is made by the development and sale of proprietary prescription drugs. The goal of the big money game in Western medicine is to develop a drug and patent it. If granted a proprietary drug patent, the developing company has the right to manufacture and market that drug without competition for a twelve-year period. During this time period, the newly patented drug can be sold for as much as the market will bear. Recently with the new Medicare reform legislations containing prescription drug coverage, the drug company lobbyist were able to successfully work into the new law that the U.S. government actually can not even negotiate drug prices. That is right. You read it correctly. The biggest customer of the pharmaceutical industry is now legally prohibited from negotiating a better price for medications they purchase in massive quantities. Can you imagine this occurring in any other industry? At the time this book is being written, the U.S. Congress was debating a change in this policy (16). The reason given to justify the twelve-year proprietary patent system is so that all of the money that is invested into the research and development of a new drug can be recouped while copy-cat companies are prevented from *stealing* ideas and competing with the company that did the initial research. In order for a company to be granted a patent the substance must be *man-made*. It can not occur naturally. If the substance can be found in nature, then nobody can *own* it, making it ineligible for a proprietary patent. The majority of the time drugs have their origin in some plant, or natural material, and are then chemically modified just enough to make it a *synthetic* compound which is eligible for patent. Therefore, naturally occurring substances having a known therapeutic application are often modified into synthetic versions so they are eligible for a proprietary patent. This process often results in a substance that is more potent per dose and faster acting. However, it also may then possess significant side effects and act as a toxin that then has to be rendered harmless and eliminated by the liver and kidneys, which requires large amounts of vitamins and minerals.

Both directly, and indirectly, the money from the development and sale of proprietary drugs is funneled back into the system funding everything from medical schools to research in the field of medicine. The Federal Drug Administration (FDA) and National Institutes of Health (NIH) approve drugs and grant research money respectively. Doctors involved in the FDA and NIH are often trained in the drug-only model of medicine, and frequently leave their positions in government agencies that regulate medicine for lucrative consulting jobs in the pharmaceutical industry. While the government helps fund staggering amounts of drug-based research and the deep pockets of the pharmaceutical industry contributes even more, how much research money is funneled to the study of vitamins, herbs, and other natural agents? The answer is not much, or now due to political and market pressures a token amount. Therefore, from a research prospective, it is simply not a fair fight. An often made argument I hear from conventional-minded physicians against using vitamins, minerals, herbs, or other natural things is there is not enough research to support their use. This is not true by the way. In my experience many conventional physicians often do not look for the research nor are many of them inclined to read it before making such statements. In the end, it is really quite simple. What is good for the pharmaceutical industry is good for organized, conventional medicine as we know it today. This is the industry which fuels the machine.

Medical school students are generally taught, whether overtly or more subtly, that the use of drugs and surgery is the only way to treat the majority of ailments and anything else is just not considered serious medicine. This mind-set is continued throughout doctors' careers as pharmaceutical sales representatives visit their offices with the goal to convince them to use the newest drugs. Through my experience, I have observed drug salespeople telling doctors to use the new drug with the fresh twelve-year patent since the older drug coming off patent *really didn't work as well as the new one anyway and had lots more side effects*. What about the previous twelve years when those same drug salespeople were telling the doctors that the old drug was the best thing since sliced bread, had little or no side effects, and was the perfect solution for a particular problem? You need to understand that when a drug patent runs out the drug goes generic; thereby, making it much less profitable for the company that developed and produced the drug originally. Other manufacturers can then manufacture a generic form of the drug and offer it to the market at a much lower cost. Therefore, it is advantageous for a pharmaceutical company to have a new drug ready when their older drug's protective patent is about to expire.

Unfortunately, it may very well be that the majority of physicians receive a great deal of their postdoctoral pharmacological education from drug company sales representatives or information provided to them from one of the major drug companies. In fact, it has been suggested by some that the majority of information absorbed by doctors while reading medical journals is from the advertisements, not the technical articles and that the advertisements in medical journals are not entirely evidence-based (17). What do you think is being advertised in medical journals anyway; vitamins and herbs? Not likely. You guessed it, drugs.

Balanced against this apparent bias against vitamins by the conservative medical authorities is the other extreme. It is true there are proponents of vitamins and nutritional supplements who make some pretty bold claims about vitamin therapy that are either not firmly supported by the scientific literature or for which the scientific studies have been taken out of context or overstated. These situations should be condemned to the same degree as the opposition. I often encourage doctors, and patients alike, to always consider the source of their information before accepting it as absolute fact. For example, just because something good or bad is stated about a vitamin on the internet does not necessarily make it true.

How should I use vitamins and other supplements?

Now that we have discussed the politics and issues affecting vitamins and nutritional supplements, we are ready to discuss what you should know about their use to help maintain and improve your health and wellness. In order to approach this issue, you must realize there is a big difference between using vitamins in order to maintain proper nutritional status versus using much larger dosages of vitamins and supplements therapeutically in order to affect a specific disease process. Using these substances therapeutically is very specific to the disorder that you are trying to help. This is beyond the scope of this book and should be done under the guidance of a nutritionally trained doctor (i.e. medical, naturopathic, chiropractic, etc.) I have, however, included a chapter in this book entitled *The Disorders* where basic therapeutic nutritional protocols are given for the most commonly occurring problems that are modifiable with the use of vitamins, supplements, or herbs. This represents an abbreviated list of disorders and protocols. For a more in-depth account of the therapeutic use of vitamins, nutrients, and herbs consider the *Encyclopedia of Natural Medicine* by Murray and Pizzorno and *Prescriptions for Natural Healing* by Balsch and Balsch (Please see the *Recommended Reading* section). While there are more comprehensive and technical books available on these subjects, they are often written for the physician. The two books listed above were written so that an average person can make sense of them.

Let us now turn to the use of vitamins and supplements for maintaining optimal health and longevity. Medical authorities have helped the government establish guidelines delineating the daily intake requirements of major vitamins and minerals. These guidelines are termed "Recommended Daily Allowances" (RDA) or "Recommended Daily Intakes" (RDI). Most people are familiar with these since the percentage of recommended daily allowance for specific nutrients contained in a serving of any packaged food is printed on the label for that food; this has been required by law for several years now. The RDAs have been under fire for years by nutritionally-minded doctors and nutritionists as being wholly inadequate. The RDAs do not represent the level of these vitamins and minerals necessary for a person to be *optimally* healthy, but rather are only slightly above the amount required by an average person not to show overt deficiency signs for a vitamin or mineral. For example, the RDA for vitamin C is 60 mg per day. In my experience, the amount most nutritionally-minded health care practitioners often suggest you should consume on a daily basis in order to be healthy is a minimum of 1,000 mg. The amount I might use therapeutically as part of treatment for a patient with a cold is anywhere from 3,000 mg to 10,000 mg per day. In other words, the RDAs are very low and certainly are not *wellness* values. When I have patients with a cold or another minor viral infection and I tell them I am going to use vitamin C as part of their treatment, they often respond something like this: *Well I'll just drink lots of orange juice*, Doc. There have been times I have been unable to prevent myself from laughing a bit as I tell them that they had better call Tropicana and have a tanker truck full of orange juice with a very big straw sent to their house since that is about how much vitamin C I am going to give them during the next week. This illustration helps them see more clearly what is meant by nutrients being used in a preventative versus a therapeutic way.

The other argument against the RDAs is that it is assumed the person in question is "average." The average person is an arbitrary, mathematical being and not a real living person. Previously in this book, I discussed the concept of people being individuals having unique needs. Some people just need higher levels of certain nutrients in order to be healthy. Vitamins and minerals are needed not as food sources but rather to act as catalysts that allow substances called enzymes to carry out needed biochemical reactions within our bodies. Without vitamins or minerals, enzymes will not work properly. When vitamin or mineral levels are too low for an individual, the enzymes will not work efficiently and the person's biochemistry and metabolism will not function optimally. This can lead to fatigue, depression, and disease. Some individuals need more of a particular vitamin or mineral in order to drive a particular enzyme harder. The reason for this may be that genetically they do not make optimal amounts of that particular enzyme or they may make a slightly incorrect (warped) version of the enzyme and therefore require more of the vitamin or mineral catalyst than the average person to achieve normal metabolism. These individuals are certainly not taken into account in the RDAs.

So what vitamins and supplements should I take on a daily basis in order to protect myself and help maintain optimal wellness and vitality?

Minimum:

1. **Multivitamin-mineral: (as directed on label)**

    A high quality multivitamin-mineral will help cover your basic needs for a broad spectrum of essential nutrients and will serve as the foundation on which the other higher doses of selected supplements may be administered. The average over-the-counter one per day multivitamin product is inadequate in my professional opinion. It is simply not possible to fit meaningful quantities of quality vitamins and minerals in one pill per day that will meet optimal daily requirements. Retail products are also often mainly designed to be sold at an attractive price, and quality is sometimes not the primary concern. Your nutritional healthcare professional is a good source of higher quality supplements available only through healthcare providers.

2. **Vitamin C: (1,000 to 3,000 mg per day)**

    Ascorbic acid plays a major role in the functioning of the body's immune system, is necessary for the formation of collagen and other tissues, and is a major antioxidant that plays a large role in the body's ability to protect itself against the effects of pollution and chemicals, reducing the risk of cancer and other major diseases.

3.   **Vitamin E: (400 to 800 IU of high-gamma mixed tocopherols per day)**

Vitamin E works as an antioxidant to reduce damage to fatty tissues in the body by inhibiting lipid peroxidation and to slow the formation of free radicals that have been shown to contribute to heart disease, cancer, and many other major diseases. Always look for a "complex" or "mixed" vitamin E supplement containing the alpha, beta, gamma and delta tocopherols rather than just alpha tocopherol. The level of gamma (listed in milligrams-mg) should roughly equal the amount of alpha (listed in International Units-IU). In other words a good balance would be a product having 400mg of gamma and 400IU of alpha tocopherol per serving. The high gamma complex vitamin E is more expensive but well worth the additional cost.

4.   **Essential Fatty Acids: (1,000 to 2,000 mg per day)**

Essential fatty acid supplements, including marine fish oils rich in omega-3 fatty acids, help to reduce cholesterol, stabilize blood sugar, reduce inflammation, help improve dryness of the skin, contribute to optimal brain function, and provide a multitude of other advantageous effects. Omega-3 fatty acids, and some of the anti-inflammatory omega-6 fatty acids, also act as mild blood thinners and anticoagulants that may have a preventative role in heart attack and stroke similar to the "baby aspirin per day" advice that is commonly given patients by physicians. However, if you are already on aspirin therapy, or a stronger anticoagulant medication, you should not use this supplement without the supervision of a knowledgeable healthcare provider. Without specific fatty acid testing, such as that available with the *Comprehensive Metabolic Profile* (discussed later in this book), it is advisable to use a balanced essential fatty acid supplement that includes both omega-3 fats, such as EPA and DHA from fish and/ or flax oil, and omega-6 fats, such as GLA and DGLA from borage, evening primrose, and black-currant seed oils. This balanced approach can help avoid an omega-6 or omega-3 dominant state in the body and an imbalanced inflammatory and immune response.

5. **Calcium: (1,500 mg per day in chelated form)**

Calcium serves as a critical nutrient in many biochemical pathways, including playing an important role in muscle and nervous system function and the building of strong bones and teeth. It also inhibits the build-up of lead in the body. Unfortunately, calcium is one of the more common nutritional deficiencies in Western developed countries. The high intake of soda has contributed to this problem by depleting calcium. I do not personally recommend the use of Tums as a calcium supplement to my patients. Calcium needs acid in order to be absorbed properly. Tums is an antacid product that does not provide an optimal environment for calcium absorption and may result in downstream digestive difficulties due to it potentially inducing low stomach acid if used consistently as a calcium supplement. Preferred calcium forms include calcium-glycinate, calcium-malate, and calcium-citrate. I do not recommend calcium-carbonate or coral-calcium.

6.   Magnesium: (750-1,000 mg per day in chelated form)

Magnesium is one of the most critical minerals in human biochemistry since it acts as a catalyst with numerous enzymes. Processed foods are depleted of magnesium and rich in sodium. The supplementation of magnesium is important in maintaining proper blood pressure, nerve and muscle function, and energy production. Magnesium also helps prevent the accumulation of aluminum in the body, a toxic element implicated in many common, degenerative neurological disorders such as Parkinson's and Alzheimer's diseases. Preferred forms of magnesium include magnesium-glycinate and magnesium-malate.

Optional:

7.   Antioxidant Formula: (as directed on label)

A quality, comprehensive antioxidant formula will have a blend of known antioxidant nutrients, such as vitamin C, vitamin E, beta-carotene, selenium, and others. These nutrients are aimed at limiting damage caused by free radicals and reducing the risk of cardiovascular disease, cancer, and other major diseases. Taking a specific antioxidant formula can fortify the levels of key nutrients already contained in a comprehensive multivitamin-mineral. Please be sure to total the levels of these individual nutrients (i.e. vitamins C, E, selenium, etc.) from all of the supplements you are taking. Do not greatly exceed the suggested levels for each individual nutrient provided in this list.

8.   Beta-Carotene: (15,000 IU per day)

When beta-carotene is consumed, it is converted to vitamin A that acts as an antioxidant, optimizes vision, helps heal skin and gastrointestinal disorders, and enhances the immune system. Taking beta-carotene is safer than taking pre-formed vitamin A when using higher dosages, particularly in people with liver disorders and those who may become pregnant.

9.   Chromium: (150 mcg per day)

Chromium is a prevalent nutritional deficiency, particularly when foods are grown in chromium deficient soil, and due to the consumption of refined carbohydrates that deplete the mineral in the body. Chromium is essential in controlling blood sugar by acting with insulin to transport sugar into the cell to be burned as energy. It is often used in the nutritional management of diabetes (See *Disorders* section). It is also involved in the synthesis of HDL (the good cholesterol) that limits your risk of cardiovascular disease. The preferred form is chromium-glycinate or chromium bis-glycinate.

10.   Co-enzyme Q-10: (30-100 mg per day)

Co-enzyme Q10 is a vitamin-like substance called ubiquinone. It acts as an important antioxidant and is a powerful immune system-enhancing nutrient. It is also involved in the production of energy and can greatly reduce fatigue in some individuals and helps protect the heart.

11. **L-Carnitine: (100 mg per day)**

This peptide transports fats into the mitochondrion of the cell to be burned as energy. It can aid in weight loss and athletic performance, reduce the risk of heart disease, and helps vitamins C and E in their antioxidant activities.

12. **L-Glutathione: (200 mg per day)**

L-Glutathione is an amino acid-derived compound which acts as a potent detoxifier of chemicals and heavy metals in the body and is critically important for the liver to be able to cleanse the blood. It serves as a very strong antioxidant, particularly for the gastrointestinal tract.

13. **See *Herb* section for suggested herbs**

14. **Consider taking a *Comprehensive Metabolic Profile* for more specific and individualized advice on your supplement program. Visit *HealthRevolution.info* for more information about this test and how to find a practitioner near you who offers this profile.**

How do I know which vitamins are good quality, and where should I buy them?

As a practitioner, I am often asked the above question. It is not an easy one to answer. Buying vitamins and supplements is a lot like buying a car. You can buy a Lexus, or you can buy a Hyundai. The quality varies significantly. This issue is even more confusing when it comes to herbal products where, unlike vitamins, the exact chemical structure of an herb often has not been standardized. Patients are frequently confused and ask themselves: *Do I purchase vitamins in the grocery store, the drug store, a health food store, on the Internet, or from my health care practitioner?* While most people have to be somewhat cost conscious, I do not advise outright buying on price alone. One thing I often ask these bargain hunters is if they really think bargain shopping is a wise idea when it comes to something as important as their health? Generally speaking, you get what you pay for. I do not feel comfortable in saying the more expensive brand is always superior, but if you are buying the fifty-five gallon drum of calcium for a few dollars down at your warehouse discount club store, you can be pretty sure it is probably not the best of supplements. You may be getting a very cheap form of the vitamin or mineral that is not easily absorbed by the body. You may be purchasing a product that is not produced to high standards, is potentially full of other unhealthy ingredients, and may not even contain the amount of the vitamin or mineral that the label claims.

As a general rule, comprehensive health food and vitamin stores carry superior brands when compared to store brands in grocery stores, chain pharmacies, and discount warehouse clubs. Look for brands that have expiration dates on them, and make sure they have not expired. Some decent quality over-the-counter brands found in health food stores and vitamin shops include: Phytopharmica, Doctor's Choice, and Solgar to name a few. Probably the best source for you to acquire high quality vitamins and minerals is through your healthcare provider. They generally carry brands available only to practitioners and are manufactured according to much higher standards. They may cost more than the cheap, over-the-counter brands, but you are getting a much better product. Some of the most common professional brands (listed alphabetically) include: Allergy Research, Biogenesis, Biotics, DaVinci Labs, Designs for Health, Metabolic Maintenance, MMS Pro, NF Formulations, Thorne, Tyler, Vital Nutrients, and others. I am the Chief Medical Officer and a formulator for Designs for Health, a nutritional supplement company that creates and manufactures products only for use under the direction of a healthcare professional, and I know the high-quality standards of design and production followed during the entire process. In general, I think the companies that serve the professional market go above and beyond what is often done in the retail marketplace. These companies provide product dating and most will provide you with an independent chemical assay of their products if requested. In the long run, buying these products on the advice of your healthcare provider may save you money since you are also benefiting from their professional advice and are more likely to be buying only what you really need for your unique situation or condition. Make sure the practitioner can give you a valid reason for what they recommend and that they provide you with exact instructions regarding dosage, frequency, and duration of usage for the supplement.

Suggested Supplement Program

Minimum:

1. Multivitamin-mineral: (as directed on label)

2. Vitamin C: (1,000 to 3,000 mg per day)

3. Vitamin E (mixed): (400 to 800 IU per day)

4. Essential Fatty Acids [omega 3 and 6 oils]: (1,000 to 2,000 mg per day)

5. Calcium: (1,500 mg per day in chelated form)

6. Magnesium: (750-1,000 mg per day in chelated form)

Optional:

7. Antioxidant Formula: (as directed on label)

8. Beta-Carotene: (15,000 IU per day)

9. Chromium: (150 mcg per day)

10. Co-enzyme Q-10: (30-100 mg per day)

11. L-Carnitine: (100-200 mg per day)

12. L-Glutathione: (200 mg per day)

13. See *Herb* section for suggested herbs

14. Consider taking a *Comprehensive Metabolic Profile* for more specific and individualized supplement advice. (*HealthyRevolution.info*)

*These nutrients levels should be taken with food in divided dosages if possible (i.e.: divide into 2-3 dosages throughout the day).

Specific References:

1. Arnold LE, DiSilvestro RA. Zinc in attention-deficit/hyperactivity disorder. J Child Adolesc Psychopharmacol. 2005 Aug;15(4):619-27.

2. Marcason W. Can dietary intervention play a part in the treatment of attention deficit and hyperactivity disorder? J Am Diet Assoc. 2005 Jul;105(7):1161-2.

3. Ryrie I, Cornah D, Van de Weyer C. Food, mood and mental health. Ment Health Today. 2006 Feb:23-6.

4. Fairfield KM, Fletcher RH. Vitamins for chronic disease prevention in adults: scientific review. Jama. 2002 Jun 19;287(23):3116-26.

5. Goh YI, Bollano E, Einarson TR, Koren G. Prenatal multivitamin supplementation and rates of congenital anomalies: a meta-analysis. J Obstet Gynaecol Can. 2006 Aug;28(8):680-9.

6. Walsh N. Multivitamins and Medicare. Fam Pract News. 2003;38.

7. Christen S, Woodall AA, Shigenaga MK, Southwell-Keely PT, Duncan MW, Ames BN. gamma-tocopherol traps mutagenic electrophiles such as NO(X) and complements alpha-tocopherol: physiological implications. Proc Natl Acad Sci U S A. 1997 Apr 1;94(7):3217-22.

8. Cooney RV, Franke AA, Harwood PJ, Hatch-Pigott V, Custer LJ, Mordan LJ. Gamma-tocopherol detoxification of nitrogen dioxide: superiority to alpha-tocopherol. Proc Natl Acad Sci U S A. 1993 Mar 1;90(5):1771-5.

9. Davey PJ, Schulz M, Gliksman M, Dobson M, Aristides M, Stephens NG. Cost-effectiveness of vitamin E therapy in the treatment of patients with angiographically proven coronary narrowing (CHAOS trial). Cambridge Heart Antioxidant Study. Am J Cardiol. 1998 Aug 15;82(4):414-7.

10. Emmert DH, Kirchner JT. The role of vitamin E in the prevention of heart disease. Arch Fam Med. 1999 Nov-Dec;8(6):537-42.

11. Olsson AG, Yuan XM. Antioxidants in the prevention of atherosclerosis. Curr Opin Lipidol. 1996 Dec;7(6):374-80.

12. Stephens NG, Parsons A, Schofield PM, Kelly F, Cheeseman K, Mitchinson MJ. Randomised controlled trial of vitamin E in patients with coronary disease: Cambridge Heart Antioxidant Study (CHAOS). Lancet. 1996 Mar 23;347(9004):781-6.

13. Lee IM, Cook NR, Gaziano JM, Gordon D, Ridker PM, Manson JE, et al. Vitamin E in the primary prevention of cardiovascular disease and cancer: the Women's Health Study: a randomized controlled trial. Jama. 2005 Jul 6;294(1):56-65.

14. Lonn E, Bosch J, Yusuf S, Sheridan P, Pogue J, Arnold JM, et al. Effects of long-term vitamin E supplementation on cardiovascular events and cancer: a randomized controlled trial. Jama. 2005 Mar 16;293(11):1338-47.

15. Eisenberg DM, Davis RB, Ettner SL, Appel S, Wilkey S, Van Rompay M, et al. Trends in alternative medicine use in the United States, 1990-1997: results of a follow-up national survey. Jama. 1998 Nov 11;280(18):1569-75.

16. Pear R. Bush Threatens Veto of Medicare Drug Bill, but a Senator is Seeking a Middle Ground. New York Times. January 12, 2007.

17. van Winkelen P, van Denderen JS, Vossen CY, Huizinga TW, Dekker FW. How evidence-based are advertisements in journals regarding the subspecialty of rheumatology? Rheumatology (Oxford). 2006 Sep;45(9):1154-7.

General References:

18. Bender D. Introduction to Nutrition and Metabolism. 3rd ed. Boca Raton: CRC Press; 2002.

19. Groff J, Gropper S. Advanced Nutrition and Human Metabolism. 3rd ed. Stamford, CT: Wadsworth; 2000.

20. Marz R. Medical Nutrition from Marz. 2nd ed. Portland: Omni-Press; 1999.

21. Shils M, Shike M, Ross A. Modern Nutrition in Health and Disease. 10th ed. Baltimore: Lippicott Williams & Wilkins; 2006.

21. Werbach M. Nutritional Influences on Illness. 2nd ed. Tarzana, CA: Third Line Press; 1993.

22. Werbach M, Moss J. Textbook of Nutritional Medicine. Tarzana, CA: Third Line Press; 1999.

Herbal Medicines

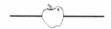

Nowhere is the rise in popularity of alternative and complimentary medicine more evident than with the astronomical increase in the use of herbs and botanical medicines. However, herbs are obviously not new and, in fact, have been with us and in use probably as long as we have inhabited the planet. There are still many historical references in today's lexicon (common vocabulary) to herbs. This clearly illustrates the importance of medicinal plants in society throughout the centuries, but most of these we are not even aware of.

One example of this historical reference to herbs is the image of witches flying on their broomsticks. We all associate this image with Halloween. Did you ever wonder where that idea came from? Well, it really came from the use of herbs. In the Middle-Ages, it is estimated that millions of women were put to death for practicing witchcraft. In reality, most of these women were just practicing herbal medicine. You see, in those days only men, and particularly the clergy, were supposed to possess any knowledge or ability that would be powerful enough to affect the status of one's health or in particular one's fertility. It was considered blasphemy for women to be involved in healing the body. However, most of the masses did not have access to male physicians or clergy for healing so they were forced to rely on traditional knowledge possessed by the community. This knowledge was usually handed down from mother to daughter. By the way, this is the origin of the saying "old wives tales". It was the passing down of knowledge in the medicinal use of plants from a mother (i.e. old wife) to her daughter (i.e. new wife). Many herbs used in those days were the alkaloid-containing herbs, such as the herb Belladonna (Deadly Nightshade), long associated with witches. Large doses of these herbs can induce hallucinations. Usually the hallucination is one of moving through the air or flying. When a woman would speak irrationally during her hallucination and start telling people she was flying, it was assumed that she was demonically possessed and a witch. On special fertility Sabbaths these herbs were actually applied directly to the very vascular cervix of a woman by putting a solid extract or paste of the herb onto the end of a broomstick and introducing it vaginally. When the hallucinations of flying ensued, the reputation of the witches flying on their broomsticks originated.

While the renewal of the mass use of herbs is a new phenomenon in Western industrialized countries, it is certainly not in other parts of the world (1). In fact, the World Health Organization estimates over 80% of the world's population does not have easy access to modern, high-tech medicine and still relies mostly on the use of regional herbal medicines for their healthcare. Unfortunately, in Western countries the use of herbs is occurring often via self-medication, without benefit of guidance by a practitioner skilled in the use of these herbs. While this is also true of vitamins, minerals, and other supplements, nowhere is there greater chance of a layperson getting into trouble than with the improper application of certain herbs. While most herbs are generally safe unless taken in extremely high dosages, make no mistake about it....herbs are *very* powerful. Fortunately though, most herbs will make you throw-up if you take large doses long before you reach a serious toxicity level.

Even in these days of genetically engineered drugs, the majority of drugs still have their origin in an herb or plant. In fact the word *drug* comes from the old English term *drogge*, which means dried plant. Drugs before the twentieth century were essentially dried and processed plants. Many modern drugs in a way still are. The pharmaceutical companies spend a great deal of money researching herbs and plants in order to study their actions so they can design drugs that mimic them. For example, the drug Valium, which is a tranquilizer and was one of the most prescribed drugs in America in the 1980's, was modeled after the herb Valerian Root, which is commonly used as a sedative and muscle relaxant. Hence the name: Valium. Of course, the pharmaceutical researchers are pretty smart, altering the active molecules from valerian and other herbs in order to make the eventual drug much stronger per milligram. This alteration makes it synthetic. This often results in toxicity and side-effects. Remember though, the pharmaceutical researchers have to make the molecule synthetic so they can obtain a 12-year exclusive proprietary patent that greatly increases its profitability. What this essentially means is that many of today's commonly taken prescription and over-the-counter drugs have an associated herb that works similarly, if not exactly, to that medicine. Using the natural herb instead of the synthetic drug is often a viable option. This is particularly true with chronic disorders where time is not of the essence. Pharmaceutical drugs generally work much faster and are more appropriate in acute situations where immediate results are imperative. I am not naive enough to suggest that all drugs can be replaced by herbs. Not by a long shot. However, in many instances, they can be. If there is an herb with the appropriate action for your condition, why not try the non-toxic, safer, and less expensive alternative first. This approach is particularly appropriate if your condition is essentially stable and you have the time to give it a try. Would you try and kill an ant hill in your yard with a nuclear device? Would you use a sledge hammer to put a thumb tack into your wall? Of course you would not. Then why use a very strong and possibly toxic treatment (i.e. drug) when a more subtle and natural treatment (i.e. herb) may do the job?

I can clearly remember fifteen or twenty years or so ago when I was in my internship. When I had a cold, I would go into local drug stores and ask the pharmacist if they had the herb Echinacea and any zinc lozenges. I knew full well they didn't have any, but it is my nature to stir the pot a bit and see what kind of reaction I get. Often the reaction was one of disbelief that I would even ask for such a thing. That is if they had actually ever heard of Echinacea and zinc lozenges. Sometimes I would be ridiculed and told things like: "What is the matter with you? That stuff doesn't really work. You need some Tylenol-Cold medication". Today you cannot go into a pharmacy without seeing rows and rows of herbs and vitamins for sale. Pharmacists attend my natural medicine seminars in droves to learn more about the proper use of herbs and supplements. Why such a change in such a short amount of time?

As was discussed earlier in the book, a lot of the reason for this change is economics. In my opinion, it is quite obvious that when conventional medicine and the pharmaceutical industry finally realized that the natural and alternative medicine craze was not just a fad, but was actually a new paradigm shift in the way the public viewed the maintenance of their health and wellness, they decided they had better get into the game. If you can't beat them, you might as well join them and share in the profits. Sharp individual pharmacists also saw this as an opportunity to actually return to the origins of their profession. It has provided them the opportunity to actually learn about the chemistry and action of these herbs and supplements so they might begin to counsel patients on their proper usages rather than just serving as highly trained pill counters and bottle fillers. The few individual pharmacists who still have privately owned community pharmacies also saw the selling of these products, as well as nutritional counseling, as an opportunity to have a new revenue source other than the dwindling reimbursement they were receiving from managed care entities and insurance companies for filling prescriptions. No matter how and why it happened, it is certainly a good thing for the general public that it has.

While it may seem as though there are so many herbs out there being talked about now that it has become very confusing to make sense of it all, you should try being a health professional who uses them medicinally. It can be even more difficult for us to stay current in this field. However, the herbs commonly used in Western developed countries make up only a minute fraction of the thousands of herbs used medicinally world-wide. Only about ten herbs make up the vast majority of herbs sold in the United States. For example, in the botanical medicine courses taught in the College of Naturopathic Medicine at the University of Bridgeport where I teach, there are hundreds of herbs in the curriculum. These still only constitute a fraction of the available herbs from around the world. While this chapter will focus on the commonly used herbs in the West, keep in mind the typical licensed naturopathic physician, other types of herbal-trained physicians, or a well trained herbalist, may use a much broader array of herbs than is commonly available over-the-counter. This allows them to be more selective and accurate in their choice of herb for a particular condition.

How do I know the quality of an herbal supplement?

The quality issue regarding herbal supplements is very much like that of vitamin and mineral supplements as was discussed in the previous chapter. There are good vitamin and mineral supplements and there are bad. With herbal supplements, it is even more difficult since the exact chemical structure and quality of a particular herb is not always a standardized issue. The quality and effectiveness of an herb depends on a great number of things such as: what exact strain of the plant was harvested, what part of the plant was used, what time of year was it harvested, how was it processed and prepared, etc. For instance, you may purchase a bottle of Echinacea capsules from a manufacturer who understands that only certain parts of the plant have any medicinal value. It is the flowering tops and roots that should be processed carefully in order to produce a high quality Echinacea. On the other hand, a bottle of Echinacea capsules may be purchased from a manufacturer who focuses more on turning a profit than in producing a quality product. As long as some form of Echinacea is in a bottle, it is legal to be sold as such. The problem arises when cheap, leftover portions (ground up stems) of the plant are used for they have limited, if any, medicinal value. This goes for all other herbs as well. In other words, bargain hunters beware! This is equally frustrating to clinicians trying to use herbal medicines since unlike with vitamins and drugs, 10 mg of one particular herbal supplement, such as St. John's wort, may not have the same strength as another. Was one a liquid tincture and the other a dried powder? Was one brand made from a certain part of the plant and the other brand another? It can be very confusing. The best strategy is to avoid the bargains. If it seems too good to be true, it probably is. Stay with reputable manufacturers. Some over-the-counter brands of herbal supplements with good reputations include: Nature's Way, Phytopharmica, Eclectic Institute, and Gaia Herbs. Better yet, consider purchasing professional-only brand, high quality herbal medicines from your healthcare practitioner by such manufacturers as: Designs for Health, Energique, Herbalists and Alchemists, Phytopharmica, Murdoch-Madaus-Schwabe (MMS-Pro), Scientific Botanicals, Thorne, Wise Woman, Aboca, and others. The superior quality of these products, along with the sound advice of your practitioner, will provide you with better results in the long-run.

What are the different forms of herbal medicines?

Herbal medicines may be purchased in different forms. They include encapsulated or tableted dry powders, alcohol or glycerol liquid extracts, solid extracts, decoctions, tea or effusions, and raw herbs. Of course, these herbal preparations can be in whole herb form or standardized to the specific amount of active component chemicals they contain. All these factors determine the potency and quality of herbal supplements. Is it any wonder why it is confusing? To clarify matters, I will explain the different types of herb forms and discuss the controversy between standardized and non-standardized herbal preparations.

The common forms of herbal supplements:

1. *Dry powders*: This form essentially represents the most basic way of preparing herbs. The plant is harvested, dried, and pulverized into a fine powder that can be put into a capsule or pressed into a tablet. This is the form many cheaper non-standardized herbal supplements come in. This is not to say, however, that all encapsulated or tableted herbs are of low quality or non-standardized.

2. *Liquid extracts*: Extraction involves taking the dried raw herb and putting it into a closed container with an extracting agent, usually alcohol or glycerol. This herb form is often referred to as a tincture. The herb (mark) and extracting agent (menstrum) can be mixed in different ratios to vary the strength of the preparation. This is why on some tincture bottles you see numbers like 1:5 printed on them. This means it has a 1:5 mark

to menstrum ratio (one part herb to five parts extracting agent). These liquid preparations can be standardized or non-standardized. Liquid extracts can be very powerful. They are particularly useful for those who hate to swallow pills, like kids. The problem is they usually taste like recycled jet fuel! An easy way to combat this is to mix them in fruit juice to mask the horrible taste.

3. *Solid extracts*: These are made a lot like liquid extracts but contain much more herb than extracting agent. This makes them less diluted, stronger, and thicker. Their consistency is much like syrup and they are often applied externally as a poultice or salve.

4. *Decoctions*: This may be the most traditional of herbal preparation methods. It has been used by cultures for thousands of years and is still how most Chinese herbals are made. It entails the harvesting of the below ground parts of a plant (i.e.: roots and rhizomes) and boiling them down in water in order to derive a liquid with components of the herb contained in it. This is much like making a liquid extract, but you are not using a chemical extracting agent like alcohol or glycerol. It uses only water and the power of boiling to make the preparation. These liquids, much like tinctures, can be very unpleasant tasting and can be masked by diluting them in juice. Some modern herbal companies are now taking decoctions and spraying them in a fine mist over the surface of a dryer in order to derive a fine powder which can then be put into tablets or capsules. While the result is a powder made from an herb that has been put in pill format, it is not a dried powdered

herb. It is made more potent by the decoction process that was used to originally derive the powder.

5. *Effusions*: These are essentially teas made by taking the above ground parts of a plant (i.e.: leaves and flowering parts) and boiling or steaming them. The resultant liquid can be consumed immediately as a tea or saved as a liquid effusion to be taken at a later date.

6. *Raw herb*: This involves simply taking part of a plant and consuming it directly. Many less technically developed cultures living in rural areas will take the roots, leaves, nuts, fruit, etc. from a plant and consume it orally or apply it externally for medicinal purposes.

The standardized vs. non-standardized herb debate:

There is a very controversial topic in herbal medicine that should be mentioned and discussed. It involves whether or not to standardize herbal supplements. Standardization essentially means there is a set and confirmed amount of one or more of the chemical components thought to be responsible for the therapeutic effect of the herb contained in the herbal preparation. This is advocated by many in the field of herbal medicine in order to create some uniformity and consistency among the various brands and forms of herbal supplements. While on the surface this seems like a wonderful idea, there are some valid arguments against all herbs succumbing to standardization. The whole idea of measuring and assuring specific amounts of individual chemicals to be contained within an herbal supplement involves looking at herbs in a very Western scientific, reductionist, and analytical way. It is rather like looking at herbs strictly as direct replacements for drugs. In other words, standardization may be seen as reducing the herb to its active chemical component only, which can then be used to help a particular symptom in the body. It is feared this may lead to giving only that component of the herb as the therapy, or at the very least may result in the spiking of some herbs with extra amounts of the active chemical ingredient or adding synthetic forms of these active ingredients.

Traditional herbalists, such as Oriental, Ayrevadic, and many of the more conservative naturopathic physicians, argue against standardization of herbs very strenuously. Their contention is herbs are more than the sum of their individual parts. Each plant has energy and healing potential inherent to it that is dependant on all the components of the herb being present. Essentially, they believe there is a synergy among all the plant's chemical constituents that is lost when the plant preparation is manipulated into a standardized format. While much of this may be true, I believe the age of standardization is here. There needs to be some rules of the game for herbal supplements now that they are being used by so many people who lack training and experience in the art of using herbal medicines clinically. The influence of chemically-based Western medicine and the pharmaceutical industry will also continue to push for chemical standardization of these products as they enter the arena and become major manufacturers of herbal products themselves. It would be ideal if access to both whole herb and standardized herbal formulas remain available, and an appreciation for the value and merit of both forms emerges among clinicians, the general public, and manufacturers.

The Big Ten:

It is certainly beyond the intended scope of this book to deliver a treatise on all the available herbs and their medicinal usage. In the *Reference* section located at the back of this book, there is a list of books that cover each herb in detail and explain its usage by clinical condition.

Listed below is a summary of ten of the most commonly used herbs in Western developed countries (listed in alphabetical order):

1.   *Black Cohosh (Actaea racemosa or Cimicifuga racemosa):*

Black cohosh has many other common names, including: black snakeroot, bugbane, mugwort, cimicifuga, macrotys, rattleroot, rattleweed, and sqaw root. The herb is commonly sold under trade names like: Remifemin, Estroven, Femtrol, and GNC Menopause. Black cohosh is a native North American herb that grows on hillsides in higher elevations. The rhizome, or underground portion, of the plant is what is used medicinally. The phytochemistry of black cohosh is fairly well known, with active constituents including: actein, 27-deoxyactein, cimicifugoside, and various flavonoid compounds. The physiological action of black cohosh is most understood for its vascular and estrogenic effects. The vascular relaxing and diuretic (to cause urination in order to lower fluid volume in the body) effects of black cohosh make it an ideal herb in the treatment of hypertension (high blood pressure). However, black cohosh is used most often for its estrogenic activity. It has been shown to bind to estrogen receptors and suppress leutinizing hormone in the body. For these reasons, it has been long reported to ease the symptoms of menopause, which are often caused by declining estrogen levels. These symptoms may include: hot flashes, sweating, headache, heart palpitation, nervousness, depression, and sleep difficulties. The herb is used extensively in Europe as a natural alternative to estrogen replacement therapy. Other reported traditional uses include its usage as an astringent, diuretic (promotes urination), anti-diarrheal, anti-inflammatory, and for snake bites.

Dosage: Depends on the form of the herb used (See manufacturers label).

Cautions: Careful monitoring of blood pressure while taking black cohosh, particularly if taking blood pressure medication simultaneously, is suggested. It is also not advisable to take this herb during pregnancy due to the possibility of higher incidents of spontaneous abortions. Women with a family or personal history of estrogen-sensitive breast cancer should avoid using this herb or use it only under the supervision of a qualified herbal healthcare professional.

2.   *Echinacea (Echinacea angustifolia/purpurea/pallida):*

Echinacea is one of the most commonly used herbs in the United States. In fact, it is reported that it was commonly used by Native Americans living in areas where it grew and was later introduced to European settlers in North America. There are several strains of this beautiful flowering plant that are commonly used. Both the below ground parts (rhizome and roots) and the above ground parts (flowers) can be used medicinally, depending on the exact species used. Some common names include: cone flower, purple cone flower, Kansas snakeroot, Missouri snake root, scurvy root, and red sunflower. There have been numerous active chemicals isolated, including: polysaccharides, flavonoids, alkylamides, essential oils, and caffeic acid. It is the essential oils in the plant that often cause a tingling sensation on your tongue when taking the herb. The plant is mainly used as an immune system stimulant. It has been demonstrated scientifically to increase the activity and mobility of infection-fighting white blood cells. For this reason, it has been reported to have anti-bacterial, anti-viral, anti-fungal, and indirect anti-neoplastic (cancer) activity. While it has been used topically to treat superficial wounds and ulcers, it is mainly used orally to treat generalized infections, including: colds, flues, upper respiratory infections, and urogenital (bladder) infections. It is also being studied in the treatment of diseases as diverse as chronic yeast infections, chronic fatigue syndrome, AIDS, and cancer. Echinacea has been studied extensively in Germany and is used by large numbers of conventional German physicians in the treatment of the common cold and many other infections.

Dosage: Depends on form of herb used (See manufacturers label).

Cautions: There is some concern that prolonged use of Echinacea can over-stimulate the immune system, although this has never been firmly established. To be on the safe side, it is not advisable to take this herb if you have an auto-immune disorder, such as: lupus, scleroderma, mixed connective tissue disorder, multiple sclerosis, etc. Usage in HIV/AIDS should be limited to research at this time until the effects on this disorder are better understood. Extremely large doses (over 1,000 times the typically used dose) has been shown to suppress the immune system in animal studies. For now, do not use excessive dosages and take for no more than four to six weeks continuously without a break of several weeks unless under direct supervision by your healthcare provider. Adverse reactions have been reported in some individuals with allergies to plants in the daisy family. Do not use during pregnancy or breast feeding.

3. *Ephedra (Ephedra sinica/nevadensis):*

Ephedra sinica, commonly known as Ma Huang, Chinese ephedra, desert tea, Brigham tea, Mexican tea, Mormon tea, joint fir, natural Ecstacy, Herbal Fen-Phen, and yellow horse, has been used medicinally for hundreds to thousands of years. The ephedra species is an evergreen branching shrub with a pine-like odor. It is found in desert and arid regions throughout the world. The medicinal parts of the plant include the seeds, stems, and roots. The herb contains potent alkaloid compounds, including ephedrine, pseudoephedrine, and nor-pseudoephedrine. These chemicals have an amphetamine-like action, making the herb a powerful stimulant. It, therefore, has been used commonly as an appetite suppressant and weight-loss aid. Due to the vasoconstrictive properties of the herb, it has been used as an allergy decongestant. Many over-the-counter drugs contain pseudoephedrine as their main component, such as Sudafed. Traditional Chinese usage includes the treatment of bronchial asthma, coughs, colds, flu, fever, chills, headaches, nasal congestion, and arthritis.

Dosage: Do not use unless under the direct supervision of a physician! Suggested labeled dosages of this herb should be strictly adhered to, and prolonged use avoided due to the strong stimulatory effects (The FDA advises individuals to consume no more than 8 mg every six hours, and no more than 24 mg daily). Some local jurisdictions have banned the use of this herb due to its misuse. You must determine if it is legal to buy and use in your local area.

Cautions: Adverse reactions include anxiety, confusion, dizziness, headache, insomnia, nervousness, and palpitations (the sensation of a pounding rapid heartbeat). There have been reports of cardiac arrhythmias, myocardial infarction (heart attack), seizures, and stroke in individuals taking large doses. Do not take with the following drugs: beta blockers, MAO inhibitors, phenothiazines, and theophylline. Do not take during pregnancy or if you have diabetes. Do not use if you suffer from high blood pressure, cardiac arrhythmias, or angina. Use this herb only under the supervision of a trained professional or rely on the more predictable OTC medications available that contain pseudoephedrine.

4.   *Garlic (Allium sativum):*

Garlic is a perennial plant in the lily family found growing all over the world. It is used both as a spice and as a medicine. The garlic plant has been extensively studied and its phytochemistry (i.e. chemical make-up) is well known. The active chemicals in the plant include alliin, diallyl disulfide, diallyl trisulfide, and others. The alliin is converted by the enzyme alliinase when the garlic clove is crushed or ground, producing the chemical allicin. Allicin is believed to be responsible for both the odor of garlic and its medicinal properties. Unfortunately, the allicin compound is not very stable and loses its effectiveness when heated or stored. This is why cooked garlic and improperly aged garlic preparations do not possess as strong a physiological effect. Garlic also contains many critical vitamins and minerals. Garlic's main effects on the body are as a blood thinner, blood fat and cholesterol reducer, anti-biotic, anti-fungal, and anti-tumor compound. Garlic is used extensively to lower cholesterol and triglycerides in blood, thereby, lowering the risk of heart and vascular diseases in general. It does so more subtly but without the side-effects and toxicity of the cholesterol-lowering drugs available on the market. The blood thinning effect of garlic also helps reduce the incidence of strokes and heart attacks. Garlic is also valuable as an anti-microbial herb and often used in gut, chronic bladder, and yeast infections. The herb has anti-inflammatory, blood sugar regulatory, immune enhancing, and possible anti-cancer effects as well. Garlic is an herb to consider taking when confronted with common infections like the cold or flu. Of course one cannot forget garlic's rich history of being used to ward off evil spirits and vampires as well.

Dosage: Dependant on source and form (See manufacturer's label). For cholesterol lowering effects consume at least 600-900 mg daily (equivalent to about 4,000 mg of fresh garlic) of a standardized product with an alliin component of at least 10 mg and an allicin potential of 4,000 mcg.

Cautions: Be careful if taking anticoagulant drugs or receiving anti-platelet therapy for a blood coagulation disorder. Advise your doctor before using garlic in these situations. Avoid use in pregnancy. May produce a garlic odor to breath and sweat if used in high dosages.

5.   *Ginger (Zingiber officinale):*

Ginger is a perennial plant that produces beautiful flowers resembling orchids when grown in the wild. It is native to southern Asia, but is now commercially cultivated in many tropical regions, including China,

Haiti, India, Nigeria, and Jamaica, with Jamaica being the major grower and exporter of the herb. The knotted-looking rhizome (root-like structure) is used for preparing ginger for medicinal applications. Ginger has been used as a spice for thousands of years and southern Asian cultures have used it in cooking for flavoring as well as for its medicinal effects. Like with many spices, it was introduced into the cooking of many cultures mainly for its medicinal effects and a taste for it was acquired over time by these populations. Ginger contains many active chemicals, including: gingerols, zingiberol, curcumene, zingibain, vitamins, and minerals. Ginger is highly anti-inflammatory and is thought to inhibit the formation of inflammatory chemicals in the body, such as prostaglandins and other ecosanoids. These anti-inflammatory properties are what make ginger ideal for treating rheumatoid arthritis, sports injuries, and sprain/strains. The anti-inflammatory properties help protect the lining of the intestines and contribute to improved intestinal health. Ginger also has anti-microbial properties beneficial for intestinal tracts in individuals with altered intestinal ecology (i.e. an imbalance in the good versus bad microbial populations within the intestinal tract). The use of ginger to treat nausea is also well known. The herb is used to treat and prevent sea and car sickness because of its antiemetic properties (stops or reduces nausea and vomiting). In addition, ginger is an antioxidant, blood thinner, mild pain reducer, and can pleasantly warm the body.

Dosage: Dependant on form used and standardization. If a dry powder is used in capsule form to treat nausea 1-2 grams is suggested, which is equivalent to approximately 10 grams of fresh ginger. For a strong anti-inflammatory effect this dosage should be doubled and spread out in divided doses. If using a standardized preparation (20% gingerols), a dosage of about 200 mg for nausea and 200 mg three times per day for inflammation is recommended.

Cautions: Ginger can inhibit platelet aggregation and prevent blood clotting. It should be used only under supervision if you have a blood-clotting disorder, are on anticoagulant drugs, or suffer from heavy menstrual flow. Remember herbs like ginkgo and garlic are also anticoagulants and can have an additive blood-thinning effect.

6.   *Ginkgo (Ginkgo biloba):*

Ginkgo is prepared from the leaves of the Ginkgo biloba tree, also known as the Maidenhair or Kew tree. The ginkgo tree is the oldest known tree species and is believed to be over 200 million years old. It is extremely resistant to pollution and insects. It is commonly found lining city streets as an ornamental tree for this reason. In Hiroshima and other regions of Japan devastated by the nuclear blasts of World War II, the ginkgo tree was the first plant to begin growing. Leaves from this tree have been used medicinally in Chinese medicine for millennia. Active components include many antioxidant flavonoids, including the flavone glycosides which ginkgo products are often standardized to. These flavonoids give ginkgo strong antioxidant, membrane stabilizing, and free-radical scavenging effects that protect cells from early destruction. This is particularly true of nerve cells. For these reasons, the herb has been historically used to treat dementia and memory loss and to improve clarity of thought and mental performance. Ginkgo may also improve blood flow to the brain by increasing the number of small blood vessels present. Modern studies do suggest this to be true, and the herb is commonly prescribed to treat senile dementia and Alzheimer's disease. Interestingly enough, the leaf of the ginkgo tree resembles a cross section of the human brain and may account for the original usage of the herb for brain-related disorders by the Chinese. The antioxidant and anticoagulatory effects also help in cases of peripheral vascular disease, stroke, and erectile dysfunction. Other reported uses include the treatment of macular degeneration, depression, allergies, PMS, dizziness, and ringing of the ears.

Dosage: Usage of standardized preparations (24% flavone glycosides) are strongly suggested when using this herb since crude dry leaf forms are difficult to predict levels of active constituents, and proper processing will assure elimination of the potentially toxic substance ginkgolic acid. For general use, including dementia, a dosage of 120-240 mg per day is suggested. Be patient! It may take from 6 up to 12 weeks to notice significant results.

Caution: Ginkgo can inhibit platelet aggregation and prevent clotting. It should be used only under supervision if you have a blood-clotting disorder, are on anticoagulant drugs, or suffer from heavy menstrual flow. Remember herbs like ginger and garlic are also anticoagulants and can have an additive blood-thinning effect.

7. ### *Ginseng (Panex ginseng/quinquefolium):*

There are several strains of ginseng commonly available, including: Panex ginseng (Chinese or Korean ginseng), Panex quinquefolium (American ginseng), and a close cousin Eleutherococcus senticosus (Siberian ginseng). Ginseng has been used and highly valued as an Oriental medicine for thousands of years. Due to over-harvesting, wild ginseng is rarely seen and most ginseng is commercially grown for medicinal use. American ginseng is the strongest and its value in Asia has forced it to the brink of extinction. The plant needs to mature for a minimum of 6 years before it possesses substantial levels of active constituents. Unfortunately, many immature plants have been rushed to market producing very low-grade preparations with doubtful therapeutic value. Active constituents are derived from the root of the plant and include various ginsenosides, flavonoids, and many vitamins (particularly B-vitamins) and minerals. Due to the notorious lack of quality control of these herbs, this is a situation of buyer beware. The best you can do is apply the strategies suggested in the section of this chapter dealing with herb quality and look for standardized versions of these herbs. Ginseng is commonly used to increase energy and stamina, as well as to help the body better cope with stress. The various chemical components of ginseng seem to posses the unique property of being able to provide equilibrium for the body. That means they can have opposite effects under different situations. For example, ginseng is often said to stimulate low functioning adrenal glands, while depressing adrenal function in those with hyper-functioning adrenal glands. In actuality, the ginseng is helping to rejuvenate the receptors in a part of the brain called the hypothalamus to more easily recognize the adrenal hormones, thereby allowing the body to better control adrenal function on its own, a process known as homeostasis. This property of an herb is referred to as an *amphoteric* effect. In other words, it can correct from either side, by lowering or raising certain messenger chemicals in the body depending on what is needed. This influence over adrenal function is thought to help the body adapt to stress and is why ginseng is often referred to as an *adaptogen*. Other amphoteric effects noted of ginseng include raising blood pressure with high doses, while lowering it with low doses, and protecting the liver in using low doses, while stressing it with high doses. Ginkgo is also used to stimulate the immune system, stabilize blood sugar, help in cases of sterility, and protect against cancer. It is often considered an overall *health tonic* in Oriental medicine.

Dosage: Highly dependant on form and quality of preparation used. General guidelines are 1-2 grams of dry ginseng root or 250-600 mg of extract daily in divided dosages.

Cautions: There are some studies suggesting the possibility of liver damage when taken in high dosages for prolonged periods. However, due to the lack of quality control and frequent incidence of adulterants being found in ginseng products, it is unclear whether this effect on the liver is due to the ginseng or an excipient (added as a preservative of for manufacturing) chemical. Use with other stimulants, such as caffeine, can result in diarrhea, palpitations, high blood pressure, insomnia, and restlessness according to some studies.

8. *Goldenseal (Hydrastis canadensis):*

Hydrastis canadensis, commonly known as goldenseal, eye root, eye balm, yellow root, Indian turmeric, and jaundice root, is a berberine-containing plant having many medicinal uses. Goldenseal, along with other plants that include Berberis vulgaris (barberry), Berberis aquifolium (Oregon grape, mahonia), and Coptis chinensis (goldthread) are very high in berberine, the main active chemical in the plant. Other chemical alkaloids responsible for the therapeutic effects of goldenseal include hydrastine, hydrastinine, canadine, candaline, and berberastine. Hydrastis canadensis was most likely given the name goldenseal due to the fact that when a stem is broken off the plant a yellow spot appears on the remaining root which has the appearance of a traditional gold wax letter seal. Goldenseal was a favorite medicine and dying agent of Native Americans and later became popular with the first European settlers in the New World. Goldenseal has been traditionally used to treat a long list of digestive disorders, diarrhea, infections, inflammation, congestion, and painful menstruation. Because of its broad spectrum of uses and effectiveness, the plant has been over-harvested for years and is now endangered. For this reason, in my clinical practice, I tend to use the other previously listed berberine-containing plants whenever possible instead of goldenseal.

Goldenseal's immune stimulating properties are what have made it popular among the lay public. It is commonly used in conjunction with other immune-stimulating herbs such as echinachea. Goldenseal has been shown to enhance the actions of macrophages, critically important cells in immune function. The herb has also been reported to increase blood flow to the spleen, thereby enhancing the functioning of this important immune-related organ. Goldenseal also possesses direct anti-bacterial, anti-fungal, and anti-parasitic properties. Naturally-minded physicians and herbalists have used goldenseal for years for its anti-microbial actions. It has been demonstrated to directly inhibit the adherence of bacteria, such as streptococci, to host cells. This property has made it a popular herb to use in cases of "strep throat". While goldenseal has a broad-spectrum affect against many micro-organisms, it does not tend to kill the beneficial bacteria that normally inhabit the human gastrointestinal tract and for this reason is preferred by many clinicians when it is compared to pharmaceutical antibiotics in the treatment of mild to moderate gastrointestinal infections. Studies have shown it is particularly effective at shortening the duration of diarrhea caused by infective agents such as: vibrio cholera, giardia, salmonella, and shigella. The herb has also been tested comparing it to aspirin and was shown to reduce fever as well or more effectively. Anti-tumor properties have also been reported; however, more study is needed to determine its effectiveness as a complimentary anti-cancer therapy. Hydrastis canadensis has also been used traditionally for gall bladder and liver disease, and for this reason has garnished the common name "jaundice root". Indeed, it appears that goldenseal does increase the flow of bile from the liver, thereby allowing the clearing of jaundice and gall bladder congestion. For this reason, it may also have an added benefit of helping the body to more adequately digest fats and detoxify.

Dosage: Highly dependant on form and quality of preparation used. General guidelines are as follows; tincture (1:5) 5-10 ml (1-2 tsp) three times per day, dried powder or capsules (4:1 dried solid extract containing 12% alkaloid content): 200-600 mg three times per day.

Cautions: There are some studies that suggest the herb can reduce the absorption of B-vitamins if taken in high quantities. For this reason, the potential side-effects of B-vitamin deficiency should be monitored, including anemia, fatigue, and nervous system degeneration with high-dose, long-term use. Goldenseal has also been shown to significantly lower the blood pressure of some individuals. There should not be a problem if dosage guidelines are adhered to. The herb should not be used during pregnancy or if taking anticoagulant, antihypertensive, beta-blocker, calcium channel blocker, or central nervous system depressant medications.

9. *St. John's Wort (Hypericum perforatum):*

Hypericum perforatum, also known as St. John's wort, Klamath weed, and devil's scourge, is a plant native to Europe and Asia. Some suggest it is also native to North America, while others insist it was brought here by the Europeans. The plant is a perennial shrub that has brilliant yellow flowers. The plant must be harvested in mid-summer and dried immediately to preserve its medicinal properties. All parts of the plant can contain medicinal constituents, which include hypericin, pseudohypericin, and various flavonoids. The proposed origin of the common name St. John's wort are many, but most believe that an observer at St. John's execution noticed the red spots on the leaves of the plant resembled the splattered blood drops resulting from his beheading. The plant has been used traditionally to treat depression, anxiety, seasonal affective disorder (SAD), insomnia, infections, and superficial wounds.

Most of the interest and media attention over the medicinal use of St. John's wort concerns the treatment of depression. Numerous clinical studies have suggested St. John's wort is better than a placebo and just as effective as many prescription anti-depressant medications, but without all of the side-effects, in the treatment of mild to moderate depression (2-4). The data was so compelling the German Commission E, which evaluates the efficacy of herbal medicines in Europe, endorsed the use of St. John's wort as a safe and reliable therapeutic treatment in the medical management of depression and anxiety (5). This bold step may have played a major role in the increased interest of the standard Western medical community in the serious study of herbal medicines of all types. How St. John's wort works has been a topic of debate for years. Some studies suggest it is an inhibitor of the enzyme *monoamine oxidase* (MAO) that can result in an increase of dopamine and serotonin, both are chemicals that can reduce anxiety and depression. Other data seems to refute St. John's wort's MAO-inhibiting action and instead suggests it acts as a selective serotonin re-uptake inhibitor (SSRI), similar to the action of common anti-depressant drugs such as Prozac, Zoloft, and Paxil. There is also evidence the herb may play a role in these disorders by inhibiting norepinephrine (a stress hormone), affecting the cell receptor affinity for GABA (a relaxing neurotransmitter in the brain), reducing other stress-related adrenal hormones, and modulating the immune system and mood via the reduction of the messenger molecule interleukin-6 (IL-6). In addition to the anti-depressive and anti-anxiety properties of St. John's wort, the herb has also been used in the treatment of bacterial and viral infections due to its effect on the immune system as well as direct anti-microbial properties. Several studies show particular effectiveness against common viruses, such as: herpes I and II, influenza A and B, Epstein-Barr, and HIV (6). Hypericum has also shown direct suppressive action against a host of bacteria, including various strains of staphylococcus, streptococcus, E-coli, pseudomonas, and others. As a topical agent, St. John's wort is beneficial in the treatment of wounds and burns due to the tannins contained in the plant, as well as its anti-bacterial and sun-blocking properties.

Dosage: Highly dependant on form and quality of preparation used. General guidelines are as follows: for depression 300 mg of standardized solid dried extract (0.3% hypericin) three times a day for 6 to 8 weeks to notice changes, tincture (1:5) 2-6 ml three times daily. *A Standardized extract is highly recommended for anti-depressant, anti-anxiety, seasonal affective disorders, and insomnia use.* For topical applications, utilize a cream or oil preparation (not typically standardized).

Cautions: Avoid alcohol and over-the-counter (OTC) cold and flu medicines when taking St. John's wort. Do not use concurrently with MAO or SSRI anti-depressant medications without notifying your doctor. *Do not use without medical supervision for severe depression.* Photosensitivity reactions have been reported in individuals taking excessive dosages. If taking high dosages for viral infections avoid exposure to strong sunlight. Do not take during pregnancy or lactation (breast feeding).

10. *Valerian Root (Valeriana officinalis):*

Valerian is a preparation from the root and rhizome of the Valeriana officinalis plant, a perennial native to North America and Europe that has small flowers in summer. The active chemical constituents include valepotriate compounds, valerenic acid, various flavonoids, and alkaloids. Historically, valerian has been used is as a sedative. Valerian's theorized mechanism of action involves the inhibition of re-uptake and the stimulation of release of gamma-aminobutyric acid (GABA), which has a suppressive effect on synaptic activity producing sedation. The German Commission E has recommended its use for restlessness and nervous sleep disturbances and as a daytime sedative for restlessness and tension (5). As a practitioner who sees more than his share of muscle tension and spasm, I cannot stress enough the value of valerian for these conditions. I have used it for many years with a high degree of success. It tends to provide a muscle-relaxing effect without causing the grogginess of prescription muscle-relaxant drugs such as Flexeril and Robaxin. Valerian is also a wonderful herb to use for mild insomnia and in most individuals does not cause a *sleep hangover* effect like many sleep medications, nor is it addictive. Valerian's sedative actions can also help those with anxiety. The effect of the herb on smooth muscle relaxation can be potentially useful in treating irritable bowel syndrome and hypertension although there have been few formal studies to date.

Dosage: Highly dependant on form and quality of preparation used. General guidelines are as follows: for insomnia 400 to 900 mg of standardized valerian extract (1.0-1.5% valtrate or 0.5% valerenic acid) 30 to 60 minutes before bedtime, for muscle relaxation: 150-300 mg of standardized dried solid extract (capsules) every 4-6 hours as needed, tincture (1:5): 3-6 ml every 4-6 hours as needed, tea: 2-3 grams (1 teaspoon) several times a day as needed.

Cautions: Valerian can have additive effects with alcohol and depressant drugs. Those with liver impairment should avoid high dosages. Do not use during pregnancy or lactation. Do not drive a motor vehicle or operate heavy equipment until you have determined your tolerance for this herb. It can cause drowsiness in sensitive individuals even at the suggested dosages.

Summary:

In summary, herbal medicines are very powerful substances that can yield wonderful clinical benefits when used properly. There are some situations where herbs can be dangerous if taken in very high dosages, particularly if taken along with prescription medications with which they have an interaction. Much is yet to be learned about herb-drug interactions since this field has not been studied on a large scale. Generally speaking though, herb usage is remarkably safe considering their therapeutic value, particularly when compared to prescription and over-the-counter drugs. When taking an herbal supplement have a reference guide handy like the ones listed in the *Recommended Reading* section at the back of this book. Use these references to read in detail about the herb you are about to take. The good quality reference guides will contain the known herb-drug interactions and any other potential safety issues pertaining to the herb. Better yet, consult a health practitioner who has been formally trained in herbal preparations. Remember to purchase high quality products, those available from your trained herbal professional, and avoid those too-good-to-be-true bargains! For more information on finding quality herbal products visit *HealthyRevolution.info*

Specific References:

1. Traditional medicine. A world survey on medicinal plants and herbs. J Ethnopharmacol. 1980 Mar;2(1):1-92.

2. Anghelescu IG, Kohnen R, Szegedi A, Klement S, Kieser M. Comparison of Hypericum extract WS 5570 and paroxetine in ongoing treatment after recovery from an episode of moderate to severe depression: results from a randomized multicenter study. Pharmacopsychiatry. 2006 Nov;39(6):213-9.

3. Szabadi E. St. John's Wort and its Active Principles in Depression and Anxiety. Br J Clin Pharmacol. 2006 Sep;62(3):377-8.

4. Clement K, Covertson CR, Johnson MJ, Dearing K. St. John's wort and the treatment of mild to moderate depression: a systematic review. Holist Nurs Pract. 2006 Jul-Aug;20(4):197-203.

5. Blumenthal M, Busse W. The Complete German Commission E Monographs: Therapeutic Guide to Herbal Medicines. 1st ed. Philadelphia: Lippincott Williams & Wilkins; 1998.

6. Darbinian-Sarkissian N, Darbinyan A, Otte J, Radhakrishnan S, Sawaya BE, Arzumanyan A, et al. p27(SJ), a novel protein in St John's Wort, that suppresses expression of HIV-1 genome. Gene Ther. 2006 Feb;13(4):288-95.

General References:

7. Bacom A. Incorporating Herbal Medicine Into Clinical Practice. Philadelphia: F.A. Davis; 2002.

8. Chevallier A. Encylopedia of Herbal Medicine. London: Dorling Kindersley; 2000.

9. Fetrow C, Avila J. Professional's Handbook of Complimentary & Alternative Medicines. Springhouse, PA: Springhouse; 1999.

10. Pizzorno J, Murray M. Textbook of Natural Medicine. 2nd ed. Edinburgh: Churchill Livingstone; 1999.

11. Robbers J, Speedie M, Tyler V. Pharmacognosy and Pharmacobiotechnology. Philadelphia: Lippicott Williams & Wilkins; 1996.

12. Werbach M, Murray M. Botanical Influences on Illness. Tarzana, CA: Third Line Press; 1994.

Lifestyles

There is no longer any doubt that the type of life you lead and everyday choices you make have a profound effect upon your overall health. This chapter provides some basic lifestyle principles that will contribute to your wellness. The information in this chapter should be considered *additions* to previously explored recommendations.

Exercise and Activity Level:

The health dangers of a sedentary lifestyle have been well documented and publicized. Statistically speaking, most significant diseases of our time, including heart disease, diabetes, high blood pressure, and many others, are much more common in populations that are sedentary (1,2). Our economy and society have changed in many ways over the past several generations resulting in the promotion of sedentary lifestyles. The technological revolution has resulted in a new economy in which the typical job environment is one of sitting in front of a computer screen and talking on the telephone the majority of the day. Historically, this is a big departure from the physically demanding occupations of old such as farming, manufacturing, and construction jobs. This same technological revolution has resulted in a shift from recreational activities involving physical activity to more passive activities, such as watching television, playing video games, and surfing the web. The migration of much of our population away from city environments where walking was a viable mode of transportation to the suburbs where automobiles are relied upon has also contributed to a sedentary lifestyle for many people.

While these factors do make it more difficult to keep our daily activity and exercise levels up, there are ways the average person can exercise more without having to schedule a time for the local gym. For instance, don't use the elevator or escalator. Take the stairs whenever possible. Walk to your mailbox instead of driving to it. Choose to walk or ride a bike whenever feasible. I bet if you think about it you can come up with instances where you could have walked or ridden your bike instead of automatically getting into your car. By attaching a simple, inexpensive device called a pedometer, to your belt, you can measure the number of steps you take in a day. This also is a great way to measure your progress in incorporating more movement and exercise into your daily life. For more information on pedometers and how to obtain one, please visit *HealthyRevolution.info*.

Taking thirty minutes or so several times a week to take a brisk walk is also well worth the effort. You will feel better physically and mentally. There is no better stress reducer than reasonable exercise. It provides you with "alone time", allowing you to think about what you want rather than just reacting to your environment like you do throughout most of the day. Of course, joining a local health club or gym is also a good idea, particularly for those individuals who live in colder climates where it is difficult to do outdoor exercise activities many months of the year. An hour commitment several times a week is all it takes. The full-service health club usually provides individuals with the ability to engage in a balance of aerobic activity (i.e. stationary bike riding, treadmills, and stair-steppers), as well as very important anaerobic activity such as light-to-moderate weight lifting (i.e. weight machines and free-weights). I have also found short-burst interval training to be effective for those who do not have a great deal of time to exercise. New research has suggested that high-intensity short bursts of activity may have a greater overall training effect than 20 to 30 minutes of low-intensity aerobic activity (3-11). Utilizing an *X-iser* high-intensity step machine can facilitate this type of time-efficient effective conditioning (see *HealthyRevolution.info* for more information on exercise programs for weight-loss and the *X-iser* trainer).

Unfortunately, many people feel intimidated about joining a gym, often due to embarrassment about their body, reluctance to look silly using equipment they are unfamiliar with, or even a reluctance to be "hit on" by the opposite sex. Health clubs have come a long way and not all are "meat-markets" full of muscle heads. My local gym is often full of people of all ages working out and helping each other whenever possible. Many clubs now cater to individuals with these types of concerns. Clubs exclusively for women have also become quite popular due to the security and greater privacy they provide. By asking around, talking with representatives from your local health clubs, and doing a little bit of investigation, you can usually figure out which clubs in your area have the kind of environment you are looking for. Most clubs also have professional athletic trainers who will fully explain and demonstrate how to use the equipment and help you develop a rational program for your fitness level. Remember, do not allow anyone to push you too hard at first. Exercise needs to be a comfortable and enjoyable experience so you'll want to continue exercising. Health club memberships do create an added monthly expense, but the investment is well worth it if you want your health to be a priority in your life. Remember, the most expensive health club membership is the one that is never used. Do not waste money paying for a membership unless you are dedicated to making exercise a part of your daily and weekly schedule and are committed to utilizing a gym.

Stress Control:

In recent years, more attention has been paid to the role stress plays in health and disease. It has been known for decades that highly stressed people, the so called type-A personalities, are more prone to certain conditions such as high blood pressure, ulcers, and heart attacks (12-16). However, it is becoming more and more apparent that stress contributes to a broad array of health problems in individuals with just about any type personality. The process of stress in the body was beautifully described by Hans Selye, M.D. during the 1950's, and our understanding of this process has grown steadily since that time. While the stress response is necessary to jump-start our nervous system's *fight or flight* reaction helping us to survive a possible threat (the stressor), it can also be a negative phenomenon if the stress remains and becomes chronic. In ages gone by, our stressors were immediate and acute, like turning a corner in the wilderness and seeing a tiger for instance. Our *fight or flight* system kicked in and we ran, climbed, or fought off the tiger, or we simply did not live to worry about it. Today stress is quite different. It is generally chronic and not resolved quickly. An example is the boss we can't stand at work who makes us angry on an ongoing basis. We can't exactly run, climb or fight our way out of that situation, without losing our jobs! Since we did not have the burst of physical energy associated with running, climbing, and fighting to blow off the stress, we end up internalizing it causing muscle tightness, ulcers, high blood pressure, and other problems.

The body's stress response primarily involves the adrenal glands. Chronically over-activated adrenal glands put out higher than normal levels of specific hormones (i.e. cortisol and the catecholamines) that over time can elevate blood sugar, blood pressure, slow thyroid function, and promote abdominal weight gain among other things. The resulting exhausted adrenal glands can also cause extreme fatigue and even increase susceptibility to diabetes, hypertension, and a multitude of other health problems.

Stress can be controlled in many ways, some of which are easy while others are more difficult. The stress response is really meant to gear up the body so it can more efficiently perform high-demand physical activity, hopefully allowing us to better cope with a threat to our survival. The physical activity itself seems to mitigate the potential damage of the stress response. Therefore, moderate exercise allows us to blow off steam on a regular basis. Keep in mind, however, that excessive exercise can actually become a stress to the body rather than a stress reliever. Remember, moderation and having fun during physical activity is the key to healthy exercise.

Consuming a diet of "junk" food and convenience foods and one lacking fresh vital foods is also stressful. However, caffeine consumption is probably the most common dietary stress put on the adrenal glands. The whole reason people feel a "jolt" from caffeine is due to adrenal gland stimulation and the initiation of the *fight or flight* response. In other words, *caffeine is stress*. Coffee and soda are the most common sources of caffeine in the Western diet. A classic example is the person who drinks a cup of coffee in the morning to wake-up. Sooner or later they are drinking two cups, and eventually they are drinking coffee throughout the day. It is very much like drug addiction where you need more and more of a substance in order to get the same "buzz". When was the last time you saw a Starbucks that was not busy? The crowds have to return to get their fix! However, as caffeine repeatedly stimulates the adrenal glands, the glands eventually fatigue and the stimulation provided by caffeine is diminished. These "coff-aholics", as I refer to them, are often eating foods lacking the B-vitamins and vitamin C necessary for adrenal gland rejuvenation and "coff-aholics" usually do not engage in beneficial relaxation. Remember, the typical American breakfast is a cup of coffee and a donut or bagel. This is hardly the breakfast of champions, particularly for the poor adrenal glands! If you want to drink coffee, I recommend decaffeinated coffee or limiting your consumption to no more than two cups per day. I mean actual cups, not the giant buckets that pass as a "cup" in today's *super-sized* world. The volume of a large coffee at Dunkin Donuts or a "vente" at Starbucks is equal to about three regular cups of coffee. I do not suggest the consumption of soda beverages at all, including diet sodas, due to the caffeine, added chemicals, and sugar or artificial sweeteners.

Finally, from a dietary perspective the repetitive eating of foods you are allergic to strongly stimulate the adrenal glands. Detection and elimination of food allergies, with the help of your nutritionally-minded physician (or as part of a *Comprehensive Metabolic Profile*), is often an important part of reducing the overall dietary stress on your system. Suggestions on the use of dietary supplements and herbs in stress management and adrenal fatigue are given in the *Disorders* section of this book.

Stress reduction techniques, such as yoga, meditation, guided imagery, prayer, and biofeedback are powerful tools. An in-depth description of these techniques is beyond the scope of this book. However, with a little research, or the help of your wellness heath-care provider, you can explore the technique that appeals to you the most. Something as simple as making sure that once or twice a day you take ten to twenty minutes and get in a room by yourself, close your eyes, and imagine yourself in a very peaceful place can be extremely helpful. Getting your mind totally off work, kids, and problems, and focusing on being on a beautiful beach with the waves breaking on the shore, or whatever makes you relax, while deep breathing can be very healthy indeed. This is called *guided imagery* and it can *re-set* your stress meter so that your stress won't accumulate over time. It is a very easy way to reduce your daily stress levels. I also recommend reading books that help put things into perspective, such as *Don't Sweat the Small Stuff.....and it's all Small Stuff* by Richard Carlson, Ph.D. Sometimes we just need a little reminder about what is really important in our lives and what is the trivial daily grind that we should not get so worked-up about.

The most difficult issues in dealing with stress reduction involve making life-altering decisions based on the stress you are experiencing. For example, if you are in an abusive unhappy relationship, have an extremely stressful or un-rewarding job, experience a long stressful commute to and from work, you may need to do some deep soul searching on whether or not to make a life change. While major changes like these are difficult emotionally and sometimes financially, if these issues are not changed and the stress continues you may never be truly healthy. What is your health and longevity worth? This is a difficult question and these are certainly difficult issues but many times dealing with these may be the key to attaining a healthier state.

Finally, getting proper rest and sleep, having fun on a regular basis, and maintaining a strong personal sense of purpose and accomplishment are also very important in reducing your stress levels.

Relaxation and Sleep:

The importance of quality and predictable rest and sleep just cannot be overstated. So many people in this modern fast-paced world are trying to cram too many things into each day. There is only so much that can be done in a twenty-four hour period. Our Western societies have never really embraced the necessity or benefits of proper rest. Hispanic cultures have always had "siestas", and others have instituted a forced day of rest where commercial activities were restricted by law. Many of these so-called *blue laws* were religiously inspired and have now been eliminated in most of the United States. While their repeal may have provided us the added freedom and convenience of being able to shop on Sundays, I wonder if it has been beneficial in the long-run. This forced some of us to rest more at least on one day a week. Our children are even falling into a busy work and activity pattern. Significantly increasing amounts of homework and parental or peer pressure to be involved in an unending number of activities in order to "stay off of the street corner and out of trouble" or to get into the best college has resulted in very stressed-out young people who do not have much of a chance to relax, have fun and just be kids. Is this really healthy? Maybe the increased incidences of children seeming to *"snap"* choosing violence at schools or the mall to express their frustrations is symbolic of our stressed-out nutritionally-deficient kids.

The physiologic processes which occur during sleep are well documented. We, as humans, have developed over millions of years to be active when the sun comes up and start winding down toward sleep when the sun goes down. Our entire hormonal circadian biorhythm is set by these light-dark cycles, and we can never be really healthy when we do not respect them. The processes of cellular tissue repair, adrenal and thyroid function, and a whole host of other processes depend on us getting adequate amounts of sleep in a predictable manner at the right time of day. Many modern day diseases, such as fibromyalgia and chronic fatigue syndrome, have been associated with sleep disturbances and resulting hormonal imbalances. For this reason, working night shifts, particularly swing shifts, is stressful to the body, resulting in a situation where you may never be as healthy as you might otherwise have been. This is another reason for making your health a priority by deciding if these types of occupational demands are worth risking your long-term health.

Taking time to get adequate relaxation and sleep is a necessity. While it is true different individuals require different amounts of sleep, most people need between 8 and 10 hours per day. What is even more important is that sleep be predictable and consistent so our bodies can adapt and find a biorhythm. Most of us tend to go to bed too late and get up either too early or too late. Working with my patients, I have found the best pattern is to go to bed by 10:00 p.m. and arise between 6:30 and 7:00 a.m. Sleeping significantly less, or more, than this can be detrimental. Sometimes people who are always tired try and "make-up for it" by sleeping longer and longer hours to no avail. They may be better off sleeping as I previously suggested, getting out of bed, and engaging in some moderate activity or exercise first-thing in the morning in natural sunlight. Walking around the block a few times first thing in the morning, before showering or eating breakfast, can be beneficial in re-setting the hormonal patterning of the body which will increase your feeling of well-being in the long-run. For more information on using techniques to help reinforce a healthy circadian hormonal rhythm consider reading *The Circadian Prescription: Get in Step with your Body's Natural Rhythms* by Dr. Sidney Baker and Karen Baar.

Purpose and Accomplishment:

People who feel they are accomplishing something in life and contributing to the *greater good* just seem happier and more content. This sense of purpose and accomplishment can be achieved through our occupation, but it can also easily be achieved through community service and raising a happy family. In my case, I feel very privileged to be able to help my patients in their quest for greater health, in teaching a new generation of doctors how to help their patients in the same manner, and in developing new nutritional products. In fact, I changed my occupation from engineer to physician because I did not feel I was helping people or contributing to the *greater good* by fooling around with machines and computers all day. In retrospect, I understand now that I was making valuable contributions in developing better medical devices, such as artificial knees, hips, and other joints for people, but I was not as fulfilled as I wanted to be. For this reason I made the tough decision to pursue a second career. For many of us a drastic step like that is not necessary. I have also experienced great joy and contentment volunteering to teach and coach youth ice hockey at my local ice rink. It has allowed me to interact with children of all ages helping them gain skills that bring enjoyment to their lives and contribute to their fitness and overall development as well rounded people. It has also been very rewarding for me to be able to write books that give people the tools they need to live healthier lives.

I think many people struggle with the issues of whether or not they are really making a difference in the world. This is particularly true as we approach middle age and start gaining a perspective that was not possible when we were young. I think this has certainly fueled the increase in volunteerism and individuals returning to school in order to pursue second careers. I see many attorneys becoming doctors, doctors becoming attorneys, engineers becoming school teachers, and the like. These people are usually highly intelligent and have invested a great deal of time, effort, and money in their original training only to pack it all in and return to school. Why on earth would they do such a thing? I think the answer is complicated. However, a search for contentment and fulfillment of purpose often heads the list. Intellectual stimulation is also a common reason for these professional changes. Often we just become bored with what we are doing and look for new challenges and horizons. While this can become a destructive behavior if we repetitively up-end our lives, I think overall for many people it is a good thing to do when done for the right reasons.

I encourage everyone to examine their lives asking themselves if they feel they are really contributing to the *greater good* and whether or not they feel fulfilled and content with their lives and accomplishments. If not, I suggest they take steps to rectify their situation. Maybe a major change will be required, such as a career switch, but more often than not it may just require a commitment to spend more time with your family or dedicate your time to a worthy cause or endeavor. Positive changes can lead to a greater self-worth and healthier lives.

Cleaning Up Your Environment:

One of the simplest things you can do to improve your health and that of your family is to clean-up your environment. This includes your home. A moderate investment in quality water and air filtration systems will pay huge health dividends. While it certainly cannot be denied that the advent of municipal water treatment has resulted in a drastically reduced risk of infectious waterborne illnesses, such as bacterial and viral diseases, it must also be realized that tap water is a potential source of chemical toxicity. The Environmental Protection Agency (EPA) has indicated the quality of tap water throughout North America has diminished significantly in the past few decades. Tap water is commonly contaminated with a variety of toxic chemicals, heavy metals, and pesticide and herbicide residues. Solid particles are commonly removed during water treatment by mixing aluminum sulfate into the water. Aluminum sulfate helps clarify the water and kills bacteria, viruses, and parasites. However, it also represents a potential source of aluminum toxicity that has been increasingly observed and linked to a variety of disorders such as Alzheimer's disease, Parkinson's disease, and ADHD (attention deficit hyperactivity disorder) (17-20). Chlorination and fluoridation are also "double-edge swords". While they can kill microbes and help eliminate dental cavities, they also provide substantial oxidative stress to the body. Chlorine can form highly toxic organochlorides known as carcinogens (cancer-causing chemicals).

The purchase of a water purifier for your home is a wise investment. While reverse osmosis or distillation systems are the best, a carbon filtration system also works fairly well when maintained properly and is less expensive. A water filter placed just before the kitchen sink is one commonly used method. Buying a large capacity system installed on the main water feed to your home may be preferable. In this way filtered water will flow to your washing machine, shower and your refrigerator's ice maker. You may be exposed to some toxic chemicals by breathing them in during a hot steamy shower. By using a water filtration system on your main water feed to you home your clothes will be cleaner and last longer, your hair will be healthier, and you will feel a big difference after showering or bathing.

The Environmental Defense Fund published a study in April 1999 which stated that more than 220 million Americans currently breathe air that is 100 times more toxic than the goals set by Congress in the late 1980's. This study quoted data from the Environmental Protection Agency (EPA) indicating that for 11 million Americans the cancer risk from their neighborhood air is currently more than 1000 times higher than previous goals set by Congress. While we cannot fully control the quality of the air we breathe, we can certainly help by improving air quality in our homes. The air in our homes, particularly in newly constructed energy efficient homes that do not *breathe*, can be full of chemicals from the off-gassing of carpets, draperies, insulation, and cleaning fluids. An investment in a quality air filtration system will not only reduce your exposure to potentially toxic chemicals but can also make life much more pleasurable by reducing the incidence of allergies and asthma. There will also be less dust, making cleaning easier!

Finally, you can reduce the toxic exposure in and around your home by refraining from using pesticides and herbicides as much as possible. Newer organic pesticides, herbicides, and cleaning fluids are now available and their usage is encouraged for your health and the long-term health of the environment. This is particularly true if you have young children who play in your yard.

Keeping it Simple:

There is the old principle: "Keep it simple, stupid" and is often referred to by its acronym *KISS*. We physicians are often taught this philosophy during our training when the professors tell us, "When you hear hoof noises think horses not zebras!" In other words, think about the common causes for a particular complaint or symptom being experienced by a patient before diagnosing them with some rare, obscure disease. I think this principle can also be useful in everyday life.

Many of us these days are so preoccupied with material possessions and keeping up with the Jones's that we put added stress on ourselves. Do we really need all that added stress by having to have the biggest house we can possibly buy, that vacation house, boat, or fancy car? Is all that stuff worth it? Is it really what should be important to us? Would we be healthier if we simplified our lives and reduced our stress, worked less, and played more? I think you know the answer to that question.

Having Fun:

A medical colleague of mine once made a statement while speaking at a symposium that fun is *something you do for the experience rather than for the outcome.* I always liked that definition and have used it with patients. My patients seem to understand that maybe they really do not engage in many *fun* activities after all. Most recreational sports we participate in are often full of competition. We are usually more preoccupied with the *outcome* rather than just enjoying the *experience.* I try and encourage my patients to have some fun every day. The stress relief from engaging in an activity which we enjoy cannot be overstated. While we do not have the freedom to engage in fun activities on work days which are as elaborate or time consuming as we can on weekends, we can usually fit in something small, such as listening to a favorite song or playing with a pet. Make it a point to engage in fun activities, particularly with those you love, on a regular basis. You will be healthier for it!

Making Your Health a Priority:

My final thoughts to you in this section will be regarding the priority you put on your health. If you are like most people your true priority is not on your health, even though you may say that it is. I cannot tell you how many patients I have seen who balk at the very idea of spending money out of their pocket on their own health maintenance. The same people who will not spend a few dollars on a bottle of quality vitamins, or to see their chiropractor on a fairly regular basis because they may have to pay for it, think nothing about going out to dinner four times a week, having a boat payment, or getting their nails done for about the same amount of money. These same people will put $800.00 cash on the counter of a veterinarian for an MRI so fast your head would spin if their dog has the slightest problem, but they would not even dream of spending that amount on a health-related test for themselves. Why is this? Well, one reason is we have been convinced erroneously over many decades that our healthcare should be totally covered by our insurance policies and, therefore, should be *free*. In no uncertain terms this is simply not true. *Bad* general healthcare or *disease-based* crisis healthcare may be covered by your insurance and is therefore almost free. Good quality wellness and preventative healthcare is NOT free! After all, why should healthcare be free? I have often heard people say healthcare is a *right*. That is a fallacy I have never really understood. Think about it, rent is not free, food is not free, shelter is not free, so why on earth would you expect healthcare to be free, or a right? Unfortunately, life does not work that way.

It is reality that people must start looking at their health insurance as nothing more than a safety net against the very high costs associated with serious illness, hospitalization, and surgery. Everyday healthcare is already not free, as is evidenced by increasing deductibles, co-pays, and declining coverage for many services. Patients must come to grips with the fact that if they really want good quality care, including preventative and wellness healthcare, they are going to have to pay something for it. This may mean doing away with some of those purely *emotional* purchases and expenditures on things we really do not need and diverting and investing some

115

funds into long-term health. Yes, those vitamins may cost some money. That organic food may be more expensive. Some office visits to your naturopath, chiropractor, nutritionist, or massage therapist may not be covered by your insurance. You have to decide if your health is worth it to you to invest in it. It is all a matter of priorities. Your health and vitality are your greatest assets. Without them nothing else matters. As the old saying goes, *You can pay me a little now or you can pay me a whole lot more later*. Unfortunately, later is just too late when it comes to your health!

Lifestyle Management

1. Exercise regularly

2. Reduce your stress level

3. Make time for relaxation and sleep

4. Maintain a sense of purpose and accomplishment

5. Clean up your environment

6. Keep it simple!

7. Make your health a priority

References:

1. Hallal PC, Victora CG, Azevedo MR, Wells JC. Adolescent physical activity and health: a systematic review. Sports Med. 2006;36(12):1019-30.

2. McGavock JM, Anderson TJ, Lewanczuk RZ. Sedentary lifestyle and antecedents of cardiovascular disease in young adults. Am J Hypertens. 2006 Jul;19(7):701-7.

3. Burgomaster KA, Hughes SC, Heigenhauser GJ, Bradwell SN, Gibala MJ. Six sessions of sprint interval training increases muscle oxidative potential and cycle endurance capacity in humans. J Appl Physiol. 2005 Jun;98(6):1985-90.

4. Chilibeck PD, Bell GJ, Farrar RP, Martin TP. Higher mitochondrial fatty acid oxidation following intermittent versus continuous endurance exercise training. Can J Physiol Pharmacol. 1998 Sep;76(9):891-4.

5. Ferguson RA, Ball D, Krustrup P, Aagaard P, Kjaer M, Sargeant AJ, et al. Muscle oxygen uptake and energy turnover during dynamic exercise at different contraction frequencies in humans. J Physiol. 2001 Oct 1;536(Pt 1):261-71.

6. Gaitanos GC, Williams C, Boobis LH, Brooks S. Human muscle metabolism during intermittent maximal exercise. J Appl Physiol. 1993 Aug;75(2):712-9.

7. Gastin PB. Energy system interaction and relative contribution during maximal exercise. Sports Med. 2001;31(10):725-41.

8. Hunter GR, Weinsier RL, Bamman MM, Larson DE. A role for high intensity exercise on energy balance and weight control. Int J Obes Relat Metab Disord. 1998 Jun;22(6):489-93.

9. Jakicic JM, Wing RR, Butler BA, Robertson RJ. Prescribing exercise in multiple short bouts versus one continuous bout: effects on adherence, cardiorespiratory fitness, and weight loss in overweight women. Int J Obes Relat Metab Disord. 1995 Dec;19(12):893-901.

10. Tabata I, Nishimura K, Kouzaki M, Hirai Y, Ogita F, Miyachi M, et al. Effects of moderate-intensity endurance and high-intensity intermittent training on anaerobic capacity and VO2max. Med Sci Sports Exerc. 1996 Oct;28(10):1327-30.

11. Tremblay A, Simoneau JA, Bouchard C. Impact of exercise intensity on body fatness and skeletal muscle metabolism. Metabolism. 1994 Jul;43(7):814-8.

12. Carroll D, Phillips AC, Hunt K, Der G. Symptoms of depression and cardiovascular reactions to acute psychological stress: Evidence from a population study. Biol Psychol. 2006 Dec 28.

13. Elsenbruch S, Lucas A, Holtmann G, Haag S, Gerken G, Riemenschneider N, et al. Public speaking stress-induced neuroendocrine responses and circulating immune cell redistribution in irritable bowel syndrome. Am J Gastroenterol. 2006 Oct;101(10):2300-7.

14. Gianaros PJ, Jennings JR, Sheu LK, Derbyshire SW, Matthews KA. Heightened functional neural activation to psychological stress covaries with exaggerated blood pressure reactivity. Hypertension. 2007 Jan;49(1):134-40.

15. Kubzansky LD, Koenen KC, Spiro A, 3rd, Vokonas PS, Sparrow D. Prospective Study of Posttraumatic Stress Disorder Symptoms and Coronary Heart Disease in the Normative Aging Study. Arch Gen Psychiatry. 2007 Jan;64(1):109-16.

16. Peters RM. The relationship of racism, chronic stress emotions, and blood pressure. J Nurs Scholarsh. 2006;38(3):234-40.

17. Kawahara M. Effects of aluminum on the nervous system and its possible link with neurodegenerative diseases. J Alzheimers Dis. 2005 Nov;8(2):171-82; discussion 209-15.

18. Mailloux RJ, Hamel R, Appanna VD. Aluminum toxicity elicits a dysfunctional TCA cycle and succinate accumulation in hepatocytes. J Biochem Mol Toxicol. 2006;20(4):198-208.

19. Rondeau V, Iron A, Letenneur L, Commenges D, Duchene F, Arveiler B, et al. Analysis of the effect of aluminum in drinking water

and transferrin C2 allele on Alzheimer's disease. Eur J Neurol. 2006 Sep;13(9):1022-5.

20. Savory J, Herman MM, Ghribi O. Mechanisms of aluminum-induced neurodegeneration in animals: Implications for Alzheimer's disease. J Alzheimers Dis. 2006 Nov-Dec;10(2-3):135-44.

Creating Your
Individualized
Nutritional Program

Today's health-minded consumer wants to eat better, take needed vitamin and mineral supplements, exercise and have a better lifestyle. The problem is determining what is right for you as an individual and figuring out how to accomplish this in the most cost-effective and efficient manner. Would you really like to know which supplements you need for your unique biochemistry and stop wasting money on all of those bottles of supplements you may or may not need? Would you like to know which foods that you may be consuming do not agree with your unique immune response and should be avoided or even eliminated from your diet? Do you know if you have a good balance of good versus bad fats, how well you detoxify external and internally-derived toxins, how well balanced your stress and neurotransmitter function is, if you are getting enough antioxidants, and if your gastrointestinal system is in balance? If you are like most individuals of course you don't. You may know you don't feel your best and lack the vitality you really desire. Now there is a scientifically-based economical way to answer all those questions and for you to know how to individualize your diet and supplement program to most effectively maximize your metabolic function and health. The answer is here in the form of an easy-to-use laboratory assessment, the *Comprehensive Metabolic Profile*, where you collect all the necessary samples in the comfort of your home.

The Comprehensive Metabolic Profile includes:

Organix™ (urine organic acids)

The Metabolic Profile starts with an Organix™ test to establish the metabolic basis of your symptoms. A simple urine specimen reveals important information about:

- **B-vitamins**: the most common vitamins needed for biochemical reactions in the body. They are involved in many critical body processes. Even modest B-vitamin insufficiencies can compromise energy production, digestion, and muscle and nerve function.

- **Cellular energy**: measuring compounds that relate most directly to how efficiently your cellular engines (mitochondria) produce energy.

- **Neural function**: especially neurotransmitters, the chemicals your nervous system requires to function and to communicate with your body. Abnormalities can be linked to symptoms of stress, mental, emotional, and behavioral problems, as well as insomnia and irritability.

- **Detoxification capability**: critical for eliminating environmental toxins and chemicals produced by your body. Brain fog, headaches, insomnia, nausea, chemical sensitivities, and a variety of chronic health problems can be related to toxicity issues.

- **Intestinal microbial overgrowth**: can lead to a wide variety of symptoms such as diarrhea, constipation, gas, bloating and even autoimmune diseases caused by bacteria, parasites, or fungi, or the toxins produced by these organisms.

Lipid Peroxides

In its efforts to produce the chemical energy necessary to power cells and fight infection, your body makes harmful chemicals called free radicals. These free radicals break down the lipid (fat) components of cell membranes forming lipid peroxides. Nutrients that are antioxidants help protect your cells against this process. The lipid peroxide test shows if you are getting enough antioxidants. High levels of lipid peroxides are associated with cancer, heart disease, stroke, and aging.

Bloodspot™ Fatty Acids*

While there is much discussion on the impact of fats on health, the positive benefits associated with "good fats" is often overlooked. Achieving the optimum balance of fats minimizes inflammation, a major risk in heart disease and cancer. A proper balance of fatty acids is also necessary for proper brain development and nervous system function. This unique test includes the AA/EPA ratio, a measure of "silent" inflammation that can lead to heart disease. In addition, this profile can show if you are consuming the right amount of beneficial omega-3 fish oils. While too little is known to be a problem, too much can also lead to problems such as increased free radical oxidation and suppression of your immune system.

Bloodspot™ IgG Food Allergies*

Researchers estimate that at least 60% of the U.S. population suffers from "hidden" food reactions. These are difficult to identify since they can occur hours or even days after consuming an offending food. Symptoms can be extraordinarily diverse, ranging from arthritis to eczema to migraines. For these reasons, I routinely consider food allergy or intolerances when evaluating health problems. The Bloodspot™ IgG Food profile tests for sensitivity to the most commonly positive foods and helps you design a diet that eliminates and/or alternates the offending foods, potentially alleviating your symptoms.

If you do not feel as well as you should and you've been told repeatedly that your standard blood tests are all normal, you should consider taking this test. Have you ever filled out a questionnaire at a nutritionist's or healthcare practitioner's office and been given a bag full of supplements that didn't seem to do anything for you? The **Comprehensive Metabolic Profile** takes the guess-work out of knowing what you *really* need in order to be healthy. This state-of-the-art laboratory assessment allows your healthcare practitioner to design a diet and supplementation program based on your individual results. The Metabolic Profile reveals nutrient imbalances like carnitine, NAC, lipoic acid, CoQ10, and antioxidants. The test can tell how efficiently B-vitamins function in your body, how well your body handles toxins, and how well your brain's neurotransmitters are functioning. Fatty acid intake can be optimized based on the results to reduce overall inflammation, the root cause of chronic illnesses such as cardiovascular disease. The Metabolic Profile will even uncover hidden digestive abnormalities and food sensitivities that have been implicated in everything from skin disorders to autoimmune disease.

Once you have completed the test through a qualified healthcare provider and sent in your samples you will receive a detailed report, interpretation guide, and custom dietary approach and supplement plan unique to your needs. By following your unique plan, you will be able to work towards optimal health and wellness in a more efficient, economical way.

Take your first step toward optimal health! Take the **Comprehensive Metabolic Profile** today by visiting *healthyrevolution.info* in order to find a healthcare practitioner near you who is familiar with this test!

*Note: The Bloodspot tests are currently not available to New York residents. However, the other sections of the profile are available.

References:

1. Bralley J, Lord R. Urinary organic acids profiling. In: Murray Pa, editor. Textbook of Natural Medicine. Edinburgh: Churchill Livingstone; 1998. p. 229 - 37.

2. Chalmers R, Lawson A. Organic acidurias due to disorders in other metabolic pathways. Organic Acids in Man. New York: Chapman and Hall; 1982. p. 405 - 8.

3. Goodwin BL, Ruthven CR, Sandler M. Gut flora and the origin of some urinary aromatic phenolic compounds. Biochem Pharmacol. 1994;47(12):2294-7.

4. Lord R, Bralley J. Organics in urine: Assessment of gut dysbiosis, nutrient deficiencies and toxemia. Nutr Pers. 1997;20(4):25-31.

5. Oen LH, Utomo H, Suyatna F, Hanafiah A, Asikin N. Plasma lipid peroxides in coronary heart disease. Int J Clin Pharmacol Ther Toxicol. 1992 Mar;30(3):77-80.

6. Orgacka H, Zbytniewski Z. [Excretion of vanillic acid and homovanillic acid and tissue distribution of catecholamines and their metabolites in mice with various levels of pigmentation]. Endokrynol Pol. 1991;42(3):471-9.

7. Sweetman L. Qualitative and quantitative analysis of organic acids in physiologic fluids for diagnosis of the organic acidurias. In: Nyhan W, editor. Abnormalities in amino acid metabolism in clinical medicine. Norwalk: Appleton-century-crofts; 1984. p. 419-53.

The Providers

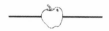

There are many healthcare providers who by using alternative and integrative medicine therapies can help you in your journey toward optimal wellness. In this chapter, you will become acquainted with the myriad of different kinds of practitioners available to you. You will gain an understanding of the generalized level of training of and common approaches used by each type of practitioner. Keep in mind there is a high degree of personal variability among practitioners within all categories.

Medical and Osteopathic Physicians

I will discuss the medical and osteopathic physician (M.D. / D.O.) first since they are the type of physician the majority of people are familiar with. The vast majority of modern osteopaths receive training identical to the M.D. and practice in the same manner. Historically, the osteopathic profession was once a separate entity from its standard medical counterpart with philosophies that were far more holistic. In fact, the osteopath was more closely aligned to chiropractic doctors. Today, however, the osteopathic profession has pretty much blended with the conventional allopathic medical approach. However, today with respect to the M.D. or D.O., the average medical physician is extremely well trained in conventional Western medicine, with little or no training in alternative medicine unless they pursued this training on their own after completing their standard education. Most practicing M.D.s and D.O.s in the United States will not be able to help you if you are seeking a non-pharmacological and non-surgical approach to your health concerns. In fact, although this is starting to change, they may even feel threatened when you bring up the subject and criticize you for your interest in alternative medicine of any type. While many medical schools are now finally introducing basic overview courses in alternative medicine, they certainly are not comprehensively training doctors in this approach. However, there are medical and osteopathic physicians who are well trained in the use of nutrients, herbal medicines, and other forms of alternative medicine. In fact, medical physicians and standard medical researchers are doing much of the highest quality research in the field of nutritional and herbal medicine. A person seeking complimentary and alternative care from a medical or osteopathic physician may find the care they receive to be significantly more expensive when compared with other healthcare providers who may be just as qualified in this approach. Whom ever you consult be sure that they have received significant training in the holistic and more natural approach. Training provided by and membership in the American College for Advancement in Medicine (ACAM; acam.org) or the International College of Integrative Medicine (ICIM; icimed.com) can help determine if your medical or osteopathic physician has received quality training in alternative medicine. Physicians who have had formal training in *"Functional Medicine"* through the Institute for Functional Medicine (IFM; functionalmedicine.org) would make an excellent choice as well.

The medical and osteopathic physician well trained in alternative medicine has the advantage of being able to truly integrate what is good about standard conventional and alternative medicine. This blending or integration of these two approaches is often referred to as *"Integrative Medicine."* The doctor can use one or both approaches, when appropriate, without the inconvenience of the patient having to see a second provider if a prescription medicine is needed as part of their treatment strategy. The other advantage has to do with the insurance industry's bias. Reimbursement for these doctor's office visits and lab tests is more common than when ordered by non-M.D. / D.O. providers. Although insurance companies do not generally cover or pay for alternative therapies, such as herbal and nutritional therapeutics, they are more inclined to pay medical or osteopathic office visits since it would not be known what was done during a particular office visit unless the insurance company requests detailed records.

Another potential consideration in using medical or osteopathic physicians lacking comprehensive training in nutritional medicine, herbal medicine, and medical acupuncture, is their overall approach. The standard physician who does not have additional training in holistic and natural approaches has fundamentally been trained in the allopathic way of thinking which by its very definition is not holistic. Some standard physicians tend to think of the body and treat the body as a collection of individual systems instead of as a whole. To them, based on their specialty, you are often a gastrointestinal tract, a cardiovascular system, or a nervous system, instead of a whole integrated person. I often see this way of thinking creep into natural medicine as well. The use of herbals by some physicians and herbalists is often an example of this kind of approach. While the prescribing clinician may understand the herbs mechanism of action, they often prescribe it very allopathically (just like a drug). Using something natural, like an herb, as a direct replacement for a drug in order to cover-up a symptom is really not a very holistic way of treating a problem. When this type of approach has been used, I have seen the true reasons and functional disorders behind the person's problems ignored while peripheral complaints are treated with natural agents. While this is certainly better than using more toxic drugs, it is still not really natural-based holistic medicine at its best.

By using the previous guidelines to find a comprehensively trained medical or osteopathic physician as it pertains to holistic healthcare, you should be able to find a really great doctor!

Chiropractic Physicians

There may be no healthcare provider harder to summarize than chiropractors. My initial clinical training was that of a doctor of chiropractic (D.C.) which has enabled me to see the many sides of the profession. Today's chiropractic physicians range from doctors who still cling to the original dogma of the profession (the root of all disease and disharmony in the body stems from an improperly functioning nervous system that is receiving interference by small misalignments along the spine called *subluxations*) to doctors who are apt to practice as primary care physicians performing extensive diagnostic examinations, laboratory testing, and prescribing detailed elaborate therapeutic interventions to include the aggressive use of vitamins, minerals, herbs, and homeopathic remedies in addition to manual therapy. In fact, the later type of chiropractor has indeed paved the road in many ways and acted as the template for many naturally-minded physicians of all types practicing today. However, most chiropractors fall somewhere in between the two extremes. While the average chiropractor is likely to suggest a few vitamins and minerals, advocate dietary changes, and even use some herbs in the course of their practice, most are mainly focused on musculoskeletal disorders such as low-back pain, neck pain, and headache. The mainstay of chiropractic treatment remains the *adjustment*, or spinal manipulation. There is no doubt that this is a powerful therapy in its own right. While it certainly can relieve many cases of back pain, neck pain, and headache, it may very well be doing more than that by removing the irritation of the sensitive nerves leaving the spinal column which control critical functions all over the body. While there is now a plethora of quality scientific studies that prove the efficacy, and even superiority, of manipulation in treating many conditions including low-back pain, the reports of manipulation having positive effects on internal disorders ranging from high blood pressure to colic have historically remained primarily anecdotal in nature and lack the research evidence to firmly back up the claims. Although controversial, there is now emerging at least some research that suggests there may be benefits of manipulation for various internal problems such as high blood pressure, asthma, and other disorders. However, more studies are needed (1-3). It is also true that just because there is not a plethora of controlled studies proving something works it does not mean beneficial affects are not occurring.

The actual origins of the chiropractic profession as we know it today date back to the late 19th century. The founder, a magnetic healer and inventor named Daniel David Palmer of Davenport, Iowa, is reported to have delivered the first adjustment to the janitor of his building curing a long-standing case of deafness. Palmer went on to form the Palmer College of Chiropractic still in existence today. He named the profession *chiropractic*, which is derived from the Greek to mean to *practice with the hands*. The profession was the only health discipline, of the many at that time, which sufficiently organized to the point of becoming a threat to standard allopathic medicine. Colleges formed throughout the country and many states licensed the profession due to pressure from people who reported miraculous success with chiropractic treatment. However, many of the early chiropractors were actually jailed for practicing medicine without a license until their states passed licensing laws. By the 1960's and 70's all states and many foreign countries had officially licensed the profession. However, in the U.S. each state delineates the scope of practice for chiropractors practicing in that state and these practice parameters continue to vary widely.

The reason I am providing this information is to illustrate the debt owed the chiropractic profession by alternative and naturally minded clinicians of all types. If chiropractors had not persisted in organizing themselves and challenging the allopathic medical establishment, the medical machine may have effectively obliterated many of the professions practicing today who utilize non-conventional therapies. The profession has paid dearly for being the pioneer in offering an alternative to standard medicine. Chiropractic became the victim of a decades-old slander and propaganda campaign by organized medicine. If you think this is a paranoid conspiracy tale, think again! In the 1980s a federal court found the American Medical Association (AMA) guilty of just such a conspiracy against the chiropractic profession, of racketeering, and in violation of the federal RICO and anti-trust statutes (Wilk vs. AMA). These laws were originally designed to prosecute organized crime! One example of the chiropractic profession leading the way in the alternative medicine revolution is that the chiropractic profession allowed the whole concept of an alternative to conventional medicine to remain in the public consciousness throughout the 1950's, 60's, 70's and 80's until the emergence of the modern natural medicine revolution. Several chiropractic colleges actually housed the only programs in naturopathic medicine in the country throughout the first half of the 20th century until enough interest was rekindled in natural medicine for independent naturopathic colleges to emerge again in the 1970's and 80's. Finally, during the past 100 years, chiropractors were the doctors continually utilizing nutrients and herbs to treat disease. Now that it is the *in thing* and many practitioners are involved in nutritional and herbal medicine, the chiropractic doctor is often overlooked. It is almost as if the chiropractor has, because of universal licensure and visibility, become too main-stream and no longer thought of as an *alternative*. I do believe this is a mistake and hope the trend does not continue.

I would recommend a chiropractor as your first choice when experiencing chronic musculoskeletal pain and would even suggest consulting with them for a second opinion on your stable chronic internal problems as well. If you are utilizing a doctor of chiropractic to help you manage your problem with nutritional and herbal therapies I suggest finding one with extensive postgraduate training in these areas. While the average chiropractic curriculum has substantially more in it regarding these therapies than the average medical school program, it is still not enough to be an expert. Ideally you may want to look for a chiropractor who also has a certification, or *diplomate*, in nutrition and/or a Masters degree in nutrition. Some letters you may see after a doctor's name who has advanced training include: DACBN (Diplomate of the American Clinical Board of Nutrition), CCN (Certified Clinical Nutritionist), CNS (Certified Nutrition Specialist) and MS (Master of Science) in nutrition.

Many nutritionally-minded chiropractors also utilize a technique called *Applied Kinesiology (A.K.)*. While this method is now also used by other types of physicians, it originated within the chiropractic profession. The doctors who are adequately trained in this technique are usually nutritionally savvy. While this system of muscle testing may seem esoteric and strange since it incorporates elements of energy and Eastern medicine, it can be very effective when performed by an adequately trained doctor who factors this technique in with other standard methods of evaluation. Since this technique cannot stand on its own, and must be combined with other methods of diagnosis, it should only be performed by a doctor and not other practitioners untrained in diagnosis. Unfortunately, there are many non-physicians, and physicians alike, who do very unskilled and altered versions of A.K. For this reason, it is suggested that you consider practitioners utilizing A.K. who have formal training and have received board certification in this method or who have at least completed a basic certification course and examination by the International College of Applied Kinesiology (ICAK). If the doctor has received a board certification in the technique, you may see the initials DICAK (Diplomate of the International College of Applied Kinesiology; icak.com) after their name. If they claim to have passed a basic certification course ask to see the certificate and make sure it is issued by the International College of Applied Kinesiology (ICAK).

Naturopaths and Naturopathic Physicians

Naturopathic doctors (N.D.) are also a difficult group to define and describe for many reasons. The main reason is the lack of standardization in training and legal recognition of naturopaths from state to state. There are many practitioners using the credentials of N.D. and calling themselves naturopathic doctors. The level of training of these individuals varies tremendously. Without beating around the bush too much, there are naturopathic doctors who are comprehensively trained in diagnosis and natural-based treatment of a broad scope of disorders, and then there are those who do not receive the training I feel merits the designation doctor. Those N.D.s who train at a Council on Naturopathic Medical Education (CNME)-accredited four-year college of naturopathic medicine of which there are only four in the United States and two in Canada, are some of the best trained doctors when it comes to diagnosing and treating a broad range of health concerns from a natural and holistic perspective and are considered primary care physicians in states that license naturopathic medicine (http://www.cnme. org). These naturopathic doctors commonly utilize herbs, nutrients, hydrotherapy, manual medicine, acupuncture, and other therapies in the treatment of disease. These practitioners are eligible for licensure in the 13 states and the District of Columbia that officially license or register naturopathic physicians and more states are being added almost every year (see *Reference* section for a complete listing of states that have enacted licensure for naturopathic physicians). In many of these states, the scope of practice for licensed naturopathic doctors is quite broad and often includes the ability to perform minor surgery and prescribe prescription medications. However, these naturopathic doctors make up the minority of practitioners calling themselves naturopaths. If you want to know if your naturopathic doctor has been trained at a four-year naturopathic school, ask him what school he graduated from and compare it to the list of CNME accredited schools provided in the *Reference* section of this book.

Many of practitioners using the N.D. credential in states without naturopathic licensure essentially received their training via mail-order and internet correspondence programs from non-accredited schools with comparatively lax entrance requirements and incomplete curriculums. Many of these naturopaths did not complete any type of formal pre-medical education before starting their program. Please do not misunderstand me. It is not that I do not believe that many of the non-licensed naturopaths are fairly knowledgeable about the use of herbs, nutrients, and other natural therapies. Many of these practitioners can help and guide patients toward greater health, and I believe they play a valuable role in their communities. The problem lies in their lack of proper training in medical diagnosis while using the title doctor. Quite simply, it is often hard to determine correct treatment for a patient when you do not possess the knowledge or legal authority to diagnose patients. These practitioners have not received significant or extensive training in physical examination, laboratory diagnosis, diagnostic imaging, differential diagnosis, and never completed a supervised clinical internship as is required in the comprehensive curriculum of accredited four-year naturopathic medical schools (please see *www.ccnh.edu/ programs* and *www.trinityschool.org* versus *www.bridgeport. edu/pages/2632.asp* and *www.bastyr.edu/academic/naturopath/ curriculum.asp*). Some of the internet correspondence schools offering a naturopathic program not accredited by the Council on Naturopathic Medical Education (CNME), or any federally recognized accrediting body, include Clayton College, Trinity College, and Central States Health University. The following is an excerpt from the Clayton College web site: *Clayton College is accredited by the American Association of Drugless Healers and the American Naturopathic Medical Accreditation Board. These are private, professional associations that offer accreditation in naturopathy and other areas of natural health. Both are **private accrediting associations** designed to meet the* *needs of non–traditional education and are **not affiliated with any government agency*** (See a list of the federally recognized regional accreditation bodies for colleges and schools in the *Resources* section of this book). Unless the graduate of these programs had other primary clinical training before completing these programs, such as M.D., D.O. or D.C., I would not consider them a physician or doctor. If you have a serious condition or are not responding to their care, I would recommend that you see a healthcare clinician with a license to diagnose. I think those trained at accredited four-year naturopathic colleges should retain the title of *naturopathic doctor* or *naturopathic physician*, while the other group of practitioners should call themselves *naturopaths*. I believe this is a workable compromise that designates only those naturopaths trained in full spectrum diagnosis and treatment as *doctors or physicians*. It is my hope that a compromise, such as the one I have suggested, can be reached so that more states will consider licensing naturopathic doctors. With the present situation as it is, some states are reluctant to enact naturopathic licensing that offers a full scope of practice, including diagnosis, since they do not want to legislate away the ability to an N.D. who has not received comprehensive training to practice in some manner. Since the majority of N.D.s in most unlicensed states did not receive comprehensive training that would meet criteria for licensure, they often successfully block the attempts of the comprehensively trained N.D.s to have licensing enacted by their sheer numbers and political activity. With the compromise suggested above, states may be able to have a comprehensive scope of practice license for *naturopathic doctors*, while allowing the *naturopaths* to continue counseling patients on general health measures but not to diagnose and treat specific diseases. This would give them similar practice rights of clinical nutritionists. In states who license naturopathic doctors, it is illegal to present yourself as an N.D. unless you have met the requirements of graduating from an accredited four-year naturopathic medical college, passing national board examinations, and attaining state licensure. If you live in a state that does not license naturopathic doctors you may still be able to find a fully trained N.D. in your area. Some naturopathic doctors practice in unlicensed states but have graduated from a CNME-accredited four year naturopathic medical school and have licensure from other states. With the information provided in this book you should now be able to ask the right questions in order to properly determine which type of naturopath you are considering seeing.

Herbalist

There are many groups of people practicing herbal medicine throughout the world. These include Western herbalists, Traditional Chinese herbalists, Ayurvedic herbalists, Native American herbalists, and other folk herbalists of all kinds. It is estimated by the World Health Organization that over 80% of the world's population use herbs as a major component of their health care (4). A detailed discussion of the state of herbal medicine is included in the earlier chapter in this book entitled *Herbs*. The following discussion will be limited to non-physician Western herbalists, who make up the majority of the practicing herbalists in the Western industrialized countries. As Dr. Michael Tierra states in his book *American Herbalism*:

"Unlike other Western countries such as Great Britain, for the last fifty years or so the practice of herbalism has been virtually outlawed throughout the United States (5). As a result, it has mostly been a maverick profession practiced by an assortment of strong-willed and eclectic individuals." While Dr. Tierra is mainly referring to laymen or non-physician herbalists it is also true that many physicians have been utilizing herbs in their practices over this period. However, they too are generally the more strong-willed and eclectic of their groups and certainly represent the minority within their respective professions.

While it is certainly true that there are many wonderfully skilled and gifted non-physician herbalists practicing today it is very difficult for me to give the reader any sound guidance in how to select a non-physician herbal practitioner. This is simply because of the lack of educational standards, non-existent official licensing laws and requirements, and overwhelming variation in the approach of these providers. Herbalists can obtain training through various methods, which include: attending herb schools, participating in correspondence herb courses and long-term apprenticeships with experienced herbalists. While many herbalists learn a great deal using these methods, it is hard to quantify and qualify exactly what is covered in these methods of training and most of the training methods lack any structured clinical internship with rigid clinical and accreditation standards. The other aspect of the training which should be considered is that it does not necessarily include any substantial training in standard medical diagnosis. Physician herbalists have the advantage of their medical, naturopathic, or chiropractic training, which includes aspects of physical examination, laboratory diagnosis, and other investigative techniques in order to arrive at a proper diagnosis. This allows for a rational selection of a treatment approach, which may very well include herbs. The non-physician herbalist does not have this advantage and is often operating on experience and clinical intuition alone or relies on a physician to pre-diagnose the patient. It must be noted though that many times the truly gifted master herbalists has a greater knowledge and level of experience in working with a broad array of herbs in the treatment of health problems than the physician who occasionally utilizes some herbal treatments as part of their vast array of therapeutic options. This clearly represents a trade-off in many cases. Great care needs to be taken when selecting an herbal coach, both their experience level and reputation must be carefully considered. For example: I would rather see an experienced, skilled master herbalist than a physician who dabbles in herbs if I was looking for an herbal approach. On the other hand, I would rather see a physician who has received substantial training in botanical medicine and utilizes it continually in their practice than someone who has taken a mail-order course and calls themselves an herbalist. If you have a chronic health condition that has not been firmly diagnosed it is advisable to see a physician of some sort for proper diagnoses. It is only after proper diagnosis that a treatment plan can be properly constructed for your specific needs.

Finally, with regard to herbalists versus physician herbalist, it should be noted their approaches to the application of herbs in treatment may be very different from one another. I spoke earlier in the book about the controversy between utilizing standardized herbal preparations versus whole herbs and about the utilization of herbs as a substitute for drugs in relieving symptoms versus utilizing herbs from a more energetic and holistic perspective. While there are certainly exceptions to what I am about to say, there is probably a tendency for the physician herbalists to utilize the former approach and the non-physician herbalists to employ the later. Much of this has to do with their training. Master herbalists, particularly those with a botany background and a strong knowledge in the growing and processing of herbs, are more concerned with the entire *feel* and *energy* of the herb than the one or two proposed active chemical ingredients. They are more likely to select an herb using more traditional methods of matching the individual patient to the many characteristics of the plant that the herb was derived from. The physician herbalist is more likely to diagnose the patient via standard medical diagnostic methodology and then select an herb based on its known biochemical actions within the body in order to affect a particular change within the person's internal biochemistry. Both approaches have merit, but they certainly are different from one another. If one approach does not yield satisfactory results, I would consider finding another practitioner who will utilize the other. If you prefer the comfort of having a physician trained in diagnosis as your provider but still favor the more traditional approach, your best bet may be to find a fully trained licensable naturopathic physician. Training at a four-year naturopathic medical school mixes diagnosis with the scientific basis and the traditional rationale in herb selection in the treatment of patients.

There is a new movement within the herbalist community attempting to standardize the herbalist's training, while respecting the various individual approaches and disciplines that come under the large umbrella of herbal medicine. The *American Herbalists Guild* (AHG; americanherbalistsguild. com) was founded in 1989 by a group of well respected master herbalists as a non-profit educational organization to represent herbalists. It is the only peer-review organization in the United States for professional herbalists specializing in the medicinal use of plants. Herbalists who are members often utilize the initials (AHG) after their name. While this designation does not actually imply that a particular course of study has been completed at this time, it does signify that the practitioner is seriously involved in the profession and is likely committed to a quality practice of herbalism. For more information on the *American Herbalists Guild* see the *Resources* section of this book.

Homeopaths

While many people think the term *homeopathic* medicine is another way of saying *holistic* or *natural* medicine, it is not at all. The use of herbs, vitamins, and other natural substances does not imply that one is practicing homeopathy per se. In fact, homeopathy is a distinct system of diagnosis and treatment whereby substances such as herbs, minerals, chemicals, and even germs are used in micro-dosages in order to heal the body's vital force. These substances, which would in some cases produce disease or illness in larger dosages, are diluted hundreds to millions of times in order to produce a *remedy*. The resultant remedy is often thought to produce the exact opposite effect in the body as compared to what the full-strength substance would. For instance, if a patient was complaining of vomiting, the homeopathic remedy selected might be one made from diluted ipecac, a substance which is often used to induce vomiting when given in undiluted strengths. This is referred to as the *law of similars*. In other words, *like cures like*. Some have drawn analogies between homeopathy and inoculations against viral diseases, since the inoculation is usually made from attenuated (weakened) viruses or viral particles which actually are known to cause the disease you are being immunized against. However, homeopathic remedies are not just attenuated or diluted substances. They are actually diluted so much that there is theoretically no longer any of the original substance used to make the remedy still present. So how does it work? That is not entirely understood, but the theory is that by shaking (called *succussing*) the remedy during each dilution you are actually exciting the water molecules used to dilute the remedy and imprinting the energy signature of the original substance into the remedy without it actually being physically present any longer. This imprinting of energy is important since homeopathy is largely based on the balancing of energy in the body.

Homeopaths believe that illness of the body is fundamentally due to a *dis-tunement* of the person's vital energy or life-force. This theory suggests that symptoms of diseases such as tissue changes and infection are nothing more than symptoms or *ultimates*, which are the ultimate manifestation of a bad *constitution* or vital force. In other words, the tissue change or infection is not actually the disease as conventional physicians would classify it. Rather, these *ultimates* represent a susceptibility of the body to the disease due to a disharmony or weakness of the innate life force. Homeopathic remedies are prescribed in order to re-tune the vital force by imparting specific energy into the body. The correct remedy for a person is one that would impart an energy that would perfectly match the person's vital energy when the patient is totally healthy. This resonance, or matching, of the energy frequency of the remedy and the vital-force is therefore given to re-set the vital force. With the advances in new areas of science, such as quantum physics, these theories no longer sound as strange as they once did. A quote by William Tiller, Ph.D., then Chairman of the Materials Science and Engineering Department at Stamford University, may have summed it up best when he said the following: "It is clear that we are going out of the age of chemical and mechanical medicine and into the age of energetic and homeopathic medicine."

The proper remedy is selected in part by the observed signs and symptoms but more so based on the personality and psychological characteristics of the individual patient. This process involves the homeopath taking very long medical histories from the patient that may involve numerous questions the patient may not consider related to the illness but are asked in an attempt to elicit as many characteristics about the patient as possible in order to select the perfect remedy. This information about the person's personality, as well as their symptoms, are cross-referenced in a homeopathic repertory, a book that contains empirical data collected from observing the effects of particular remedies on thousands of patients throughout the years in order to arrive at a proper remedy prescription for the patient.

This form of medicine was first introduced by the German physician Samuel Hahnemann in his treatise of homeopathy called *The Orgenon of the Healing Art*, and later interpreted by the American homeopath James Tyler Kent in his book *Lectures on Homeopathic Philosophy* (6,7). Homeopathic principles spread quickly from Germany to the rest of Europe and America. At the turn of the 20th century homeopathy was at its zenith with 18 homeopathic medical schools, over 100 homeopathic hospitals, thousands of pharmacies carrying homeopathic remedies, and over 25% of medical physicians considering themselves homeopaths in the United States alone. When the political and financial tides of the industrial revolution favored the full-strength chemical model of medicine, which offered rapid symptom suppressing results, homeopathy eventually fell out of favor with most medical physicians. It is now making a large resurgence due to the better appreciation and awareness of the limitations of pharmaceutical-based medicine.

While many of the *classically trained* homeopaths are medical doctors, others such as naturopaths and chiropractors may elect to receive *classic* training as well. (Many of the very small percentage of medical physicians who are practicing homeopaths use the designation of M.D. (H), with the H signifying that they are a homeopath). It must be pointed out, however, that many doctors and laymen alike are now utilizing homeopathic remedies but usually not in a *classic* manner. Rather than basing the remedy selection on exhaustive individualized research into the patient's characteristics and symptoms, such as a *classically* trained homeopath would do, the remedies are used in an *off the shelf* manner in order to treat one specific symptom. This is never done in *classic* homeopathy and is actually thought to be contradictory to it. This symptom-selected remedy approach is thought to mask the symptom just as a drug would, thereby driving the problem deeper by removing the outward sign of *dis-tunement* of the vital force without actually fixing it. Also for this reason, the use of an un-diluted drug or herb is never used by *classic* homeopaths. The use of remedies with multiple substances contained in them, as well as the utilization of repeated doses of the same remedy, are also discouraged by *classic* homeopaths and this approach is often referred to as false or *pseudo-homeopathy*. However, this model of homeopathy, or *pseudo-homeopathy*, has become the rule rather than the exception. While the use of specific remedies for a specific symptom, such as arnica for bruises and trauma, may very well help your condition, if you are seriously considering trying the homeopathic approach to a complicated chronic health problem I would suggest contacting the homeopathic organizations listed in the *Resource* section of this book in order to secure a referral to a *classically* trained homeopathic clinician in your area.

Nutritionists & Dieticians

The general public is often confused by the roles of nutritionists and dieticians. Don't worry, so are most physicians! The average thoughts of what a nutritionist or dietician does involves the idea of counseling people on how to eat healthier or eat in a specific way for a particular medical problem. While this is certainly true, there is a distinction that must be made between the typical nutritional/dietary counseling by a registered dietician (R.D.) versus clinical or therapeutic nutrition as practiced by a certified clinical nutritionist or certified nutritional specialists (C.C.N. / C.N.S.). The registered dietician (R.D.) is more likely not to aggressively use nutritional supplements or to deviate from the more conservative, and many would say flawed, stock dietary advice that has been doled out by the conventional medical establishment over the past several decades that has resulted in more obesity and chronic disease. However, there are certainly many progressive registered dieticians as well. While the clinical nutritionist (C.C.N. / C.N.S.) practicing *therapeutic* nutrition may also discuss issues related to eating patterns, they will also generally be much more aggressive in using dietary supplements. Using the latest nutritional studies published, they will often use fairly large therapeutic levels of vitamins, minerals, amino acids, and even some herbs, in order to help a person with a particular disorder or disease. While both providers serve a very valuable role in the healthcare delivery system the distinction between them really needs to be clarified and understood. It must also be stressed that neither of these providers has the scope of practice, according to state laws, to diagnose or provide primary treatment for a specific disease. They are supposed to use nutritional therapy to help patients in optimizing their general health or support the primary treatment being provided by the patient's doctor. If you are seeing a primary care physician who is not particularly versed in complimentary medicine and nutritional therapy it is often beneficial for you to also utilize the services of a well trained, and experienced clinical nutritionist or progressive dietician.

Acupuncturists and Oriental Medicine Doctors

Any discussion of acupuncture and oriental medicine is a difficult task in Western countries since these ancient modes of healthcare are based on entirely different cultural beliefs than those in Western countries. Westerners are schooled and raised in a culture that only accepts the reductionist scientific model, which in clinical applications is based on the identification of the physical and biochemical pathways by which processes occur within the body, and by which something may therapeutically affect the body. Oriental medicine is not based on these principles but is based more on the accumulated empirical observation of patients by oriental practitioners over thousands of years and on theories of the flow of energy and *life-force* within the body, including a balancing of the competitive energy forces of *Yin* and *Yang*. The whole subject of proper energy flow, and its health ramifications, within the body has always been a difficult subject for Western medical scientists to comprehend. Since these theories and principles are very hard to quantify objectively in a laboratory, they have been traditionally rejected as *hog wash* by Western medicine. This, however, is changing rapidly and bio-energetic medicine is now one of the most cutting-edge areas in medical research along with genetic engineering. Many Western scientists are predicting that the further understanding of how energy is created, resonates, and flows within individual cells and throughout the body will represent the next great frontier of medicine.

Chinese medicine has been practiced for over 5,000 years and was originally rooted in numerology and astrology. Since its inception, Chinese medicine has been growing and evolving. It pre-dates Budism and Taoism, although some of those concepts have been woven through the principles of the Oriental medicine art. One concept of Taoism in Chinese medicine is the thought that there is no real *cause* and *effect* for things. This is consistent with Taoist thinking that states things just are, with all things being pre-determined and intertwined. In Chinese medicine, treating a disease is too late. It is compared by Chinese medicine practitioners to waiting until you are thirsty to start digging a well. The goal in Chinese medicine is to keep the patient balanced and healthy so disease does not ensue. Traditionally, Chinese physicians are paid only if a patient in their care does NOT get sick. A regular fee is commonly paid the oriental physician by a family as long as everyone stays healthy. You can think of this as a strange version of the first insurance policy ever written, except in the West we do not get to stop paying our premiums once we get sick and while receiving medical care, which is the case in oriental medicine. It is exactly the reverse in Western medicine where you pay more once you become sick in order to be cured. The sicker you become the more you pay and the more money is generated within the medical system. Where is the incentive in such a system to keep people well and when ill get them better as quickly as possible?

While acupuncture was the first modality of oriental medicine to gain a great deal of attention in the West, it only represents a portion of the vast array of therapies within Chinese or Oriental medicine. Acupuncture involves the insertion of very thin needles into very specific spots on the body in an attempt to balance the flow of energy (or *"Chi /Qi"*, as the Chinese refer to it) throughout the body. The needle stimulation is used in order to either promote energy flow that is blocked or reduce the amount of excess energy flowing in a specific area of the body. Recently, the use of very fine streams of electrical current or lasers have been applied to provide the stimulation rather than using needles. This has made acupuncture much more attractive to many of those who have a strong aversion to needles, even though a well trained practitioner can perform acupuncture with little or no pain at all associated with needle insertion and removal. While acupuncture has been used by master practitioners of Oriental medicine for thousands of years to treat internal disorders of all types, its use in the West is usually limited to reducing pain, particularly the pain associated with musculoskeletal problems. It has also gained some acceptance in treating addictions such as smoking and overeating. Acupuncture has been limited in the West due to the fact that acupuncture training takes a very long time and is usually done under the apprenticeship of a master practitioner. The treatment of internal organ disorders is usually taught by the mentor once absolute mastery of the less complicated pain-blocking and musculoskeletal techniques has been attained by the student. Most Western-trained acupuncturists have not attained this level of expertise and have not received the comprehensive training needed to treat the more complicated internal-based disorders.

Acupuncture is practiced by various kinds of providers in the West. It is regulated differently from state to state with some states requiring a pre-determined amount of training and official licensure and others having none, or very little, regulation. Acupuncture is commonly practiced by licensed acupuncturists (L.Ac) and oriental medical doctors (O.M.D.). Postgraduate acupuncture training is also available for medical, chiropractic, and naturopathic doctors. If you decide to try acupuncture, make sure you find a practitioner who has been properly trained.

Physician basic training courses should be a minimum of 100 to 300 hours, while typical licensed acupuncturists have substantially more training than this. If you decide to try acupuncture make sure not only that the practitioner is adequately trained but that the facility is very clean and a brand new wrapped sterile needle is used for each insertion.

Many acupuncturists, and virtually all Oriental medical doctors, utilize Chinese herbal preparations in order to correct energy flow and provide overall balance within the systems of the body. The West began using Chinese medical herbs over 1,000 years ago. As the *spice trade* developed between the West and China, traders sought herbs to cure the great plagues of Europe. However, Chinese herbalism differs substantially from Western herbalism in that a larger variation of herbs is used than is customary in Western herbalism. Chinese herbalists also rarely utilize just one or two herbs. *Whole* herbs are used that are not standardized to the level of any one particular active ingredient as is the trend in Western herbalism. Typical Chinese herbal medicines contain a *"master or emperor"* herb and many other *"helper or slave"* herbs in combination within an herbal preparation. This is done in order to balance out the herbal medicine to accomplish the exact effects desired by the herbalist.

While Chinese/Oriental medicine takes an entirely different approach to diagnosis and treatment, and even has a totally different concept of the various organs of the body, it appears that practitioners of Oriental medicine often arrive at the same diagnosis as one another for a given complaint. This gives the Oriental medical approach a high degree of inter-examiner reliability. This essentially means these practitioners are consistent with one another. A particular Oriental medical diagnosis also tends to consistently correlate with a particular Western medical diagnosis. This is very important since both approaches are validated even though they are entirely different from one another. In other words, there is more than one way to *skin a cat* when it comes to diagnosis and treatment of human ailments. Remember, while we in the West tend to look at our high-tech, scientific-based medicine as the most valid and learned medicine system, this system as we know it has only been in existence for little more than 100 years. The Chinese system of medicine has been in existence, and has been refined and perfected, for thousands of years. Things without value or validity do not tend to stick around and flourish for thousands of years!

Massage Therapists

Who doesn't like a good massage? I think most people who have had a professional massage by a trained therapist (R.M.T., L.M.T.) would agree it can be a very relaxing and often therapeutic experience. Massage has many benefits ranging from actual reduction in muscle tightness to just plain old feeling better due to you taking some time and pampering yourself. The benefits of actually dedicating a 30 or 60 minute block of time in your busy life for yourself, combined with the action of having someone actually lay hands on you in a caring way cannot be overstated. Massage comes in various styles ranging from Swedish massage, which is "light" and relaxing, to Shiatsu and other deep forms of massage or pressure application meant to more aggressively treat particular muscular problem areas. Some therapists also train in advanced therapeutic techniques such as Myofascial Release, St. John's technique, and others, in an attempt to treat various myofascial pain syndromes or *trigger points*. If you are looking for a relaxing massage, these deeper methods may not be for you. However, if you have specific muscular problems, it may just fit the bill. It is up to you to communicate with your massage therapist clearly in order to convey what your exact goals are for your massage. It should be noted that if your muscular or joint problem seems severe, or if it is not steadily improving over time, a consultation with a licensed medical, chiropractic, or naturopathic doctor is suggested for proper diagnosis.

The training requirements and laws governing licensure for massage therapists vary widely from state to state. Some states require comprehensive training and examination, while others require none. The therapeutic massage profession has faced political difficulties, and indeed public perception problems, over the association of *massage* as a ruse for sex for hire. The so-called *massage parlor* often comes to mind. While both political and public perception problems have diminished substantially over the past decade or two, many highly ethical, well trained massage therapists still experience frustration due to the difficulty in shaking this association. In this regard, the prospective patient needs to trust their instincts. It is usually pretty obvious who the legitimate therapeutic massage therapists are based on location, office environment, and professionalism of the therapist. Always ask to see a therapist's license or registration to practice and consider utilizing a therapist based on personal referral.

My final point regarding massage therapists is that their training, and legal scope of practice, is limited to massage. Massage therapists receive no extensive training in the medical sciences or diagnosis, nor do they have the legal authority to diagnose disease like a medical, osteopathic, chiropractic, or licensed naturopathic doctor. Unfortunately, I have found it not uncommon for some massage therapists to over-step their boundaries in this regard. I have had patients who were told by massage therapists that they had all sorts of problems ranging from systemic yeast infections, to calcium deficiencies, to liver problems all without the benefit of any form of objective diagnosis. Numerous colleagues have reported similar experiences to me as well. Some therapists dole out advice on the taking of vitamin and herbal supplements as well. I am not referring to giving advice to take a multivitamin or other basic and common sense recommendations. I am talking about massage therapists suggesting specific supplements for particular health problems. Unless the massage therapist has additional legitimate training and credentials in clinical nutrition, I would suggest seeing a qualified practitioner for nutritional or herbal guidance.

The latest trend for massage therapists is to emerge from a weekend seminar or two as *healers*. Many study an esoteric form of hands-off energy therapy called *Reiki*. While I am not passing ultimate judgment on this technique and I am not a person who believes there is no potential benefit to various forms of *energy-based* therapy, this trend troubles me a great deal. Once you read the section below on *healers and intuitives* I think you will have a better understanding of my thoughts in this regard. In any event, in my opinion, this sub-set of massage therapists are over-stepping their bounds in regard to their training and legal authority in attempting to diagnose and treat patients for a whole host of real or fictional health conditions.

It is my advice that you avoid this type of therapist. Instead find a well trained massage therapist who confines themselves to the practice of massage and with whom you can have a good rapport.

Healers and Intuitives

As you undoubtedly can tell from my comments about massage therapists who engage in *energy healing* and other intuitive forms of therapy, I have some reservations about this approach. While I have personally experienced dramatic responses to energetic approaches by well trained clinicians, such as acupuncturists, homeopaths and doctors utilizing applied kinesiology, I have my doubts as to the validity of a great deal of what is done in the name of *healing, energy medicine*, and *intuition*. This is not to be interpreted as skepticism over the power of the mind and positive thoughts in the healing process. However, it is entirely a different matter when considering *healers* and *intuitives* as diagnosticians and primary healthcare providers. While techniques such as acupuncture and applied kinesiology utilize energy-based concepts in some therapy and diagnosis, they are not entirely based on it. These techniques are also generally employed by clinicians who have advanced training and a license to diagnose. What this means is they often combine these approaches with standard science-based examination and diagnostic techniques in their overall patient

156

assessment and management. This provides me with a much higher level of comfort. Unfortunately, much of the supposed *healing* and *seeing* or s*ensing of disease* is being done by laypeople and other minimally trained, or untrained, individuals. This is particularly dangerous if the patient is basing health-care decisions solely on their advice, particularly if they are foregoing more proven approaches in order to pursue a cure through a *healer*.

I do think we have a very limited knowledge and view of the workings of the human body. We are indeed more than the sum of our biochemistry, and Western medicine relies on a very narrow minded paradigm based on reductionism. The Chinese have always considered the proper flow of energy in and around the body as of extreme importance in their effective and ancient form of medicine. I believe the understanding of energy patterns and flow in and around the body will be one of the next great horizons in medical understanding and treatment. Unfortunately, the understanding and application of these concepts are in the infantile stages. All the concepts in energy-medicine are very hard to measure, quantify, prove, or disprove with current technology. For this reason alone it is a hard subject to objectively consider and evaluate. Hopefully our understanding of these phenomena will grow with our ability to monitor and tests theories. However, until the time comes when a greater understanding of this approach is at hand, I believe it should be used as no more than an additional or *complimentary* therapy in health care and certainly should not be used in place of other better understood and tested diagnostic and treatment approaches.

157

References:

1. Leboeuf-Yde C, Pedersen EN, Bryner P, Cosman D, Hayek R, Meeker WC, et al. Self-reported nonmusculoskeletal responses to chiropractic intervention: a multination survey. J Manipulative Physiol Ther. 2005 Jun;28(5):294-302; discussion 65-6.

2. Nielsen NH, Bronfort G, Bendix T, Madsen F, Weeke B. Chronic asthma and chiropractic spinal manipulation: a randomized clinical trial. Clin Exp Allergy. 1995 Jan;25(1):80-8.

3. Plaugher G, Long CR, Alcantara J, Silveus AD, Wood H, Lotun K, et al. Practice-based randomized controlled-comparison clinical trial of chiropractic adjustments and brief massage treatment at sites of subluxation in subjects with essential hypertension: pilot study. J Manipulative Physiol Ther. 2002 May;25(4):221-39.

4. Traditional medicine. A world survey on medicinal plants and herbs. J Ethnopharmacol. 1980 Mar;2(1):1-92.

5. Tierra M. American Herbalism: Essays on Herbs and Herbalism. Berkley: Crossing Press; 1992.

6. Hahnemann S. Organon of the Medical Art. Redmond, WA: Birdcage Books; 1996 (originally published 1842).

7. Kent J. Lectures on Homeopathic Philosophy. Berkley: North Atlantic Books 1979 (orig. published 1900).

The New Paradigm: "The New Medicine"

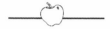

So far in this book I am sure I have conveyed a sense of disenchantment with the overall approach and focus of standard or conventional Western medicine. It is plainly too focused on overt pathology or sickness and not nearly focused enough on optimal health and wellness. This approach and philosophy has resulted in a health care system that often refuses to intervene until the patient's health problem is fairly severe and they are in need of *crisis* management. It is also obvious that many members of the general public feel similarly, largely accounting for the meteoric rise in *alternative* approaches to health management that more aggressively promote prevention of disease in the first place and the pursuit of optimal wellness (1). I have partially covered the political aspects of conventional Western medicine that seem to mandate the advocacy of prescription and over-the-counter synthetic medications and surgery as the only answers while historically promoting the active suppression of more *natural* and preventive approaches. However, things are changing.

The most promising and striking example of this underlying current of change, that very well may represent a potential paradigm shift in how doctors think, is the rise in a phenomena referred to by many names: functional medicine, metabolic medicine, comprehensive medicine, and integrative medicine. By any name, it is a movement within the scientific-based health care community, including medical, chiropractic, and naturopathic doctors, as well as other clinicians, that has struck a nerve even with healthcare providers who have previously felt uncomfortable with the whole thought of non-conventional approaches. There has even been significant interest from many nationally renowned physicians from the hallowed ivy-covered towers and halls of academic allopathic medicine. The reasons for this are many, but leading the list is the fact it makes so much sense. This new medicine also packages this emerging paradigm of thinking into a very scientifically valid and research-based body of knowledge that provides a level of credibility that no other new or *alternative* approach has ever enjoyed.

For instance, the movement of *Functional Medicine* is defined as "A patient-centered, science-based health care that identifies and addresses underlying biochemical, physiological, environmental and psychological factors to reverse disease progression and enhance vitality." This new *functional* approach is further summarized exquisitely by Dr. Michael Lyon in his book *Healing the Hyper Active Brain Through the New Science of Functional Medicine* when he states, "Most medical treatments are considered satisfactory if they simply reduce or eliminate the symptoms of a disease, or even just alter the results of a laboratory test. In many instances, little consideration is given for the overall quality of a patient's life or their ability to function as a productive member of society. Rather than depending on single, powerful treatments such as drugs or surgery, Functional Medicine relies more upon intelligent and individualized combinations of treatments or protocols (2)." Dr. Lyon goes on to say, "To be considered as consistent with the principles of Functional Medicine, a treatment method must fulfill four important criteria. It must:

1. Carry no risk of doing harm and should be free of unpleasant side-effects.

2. Improve symptoms as well as the overall function and quality of life.

3. Help to correct the underlying causes of the disorder.

4. Improve the long-term prognosis for the patient.

In order for physicians to be comfortable with this approach, it is often necessary for them to forget a great deal about how they were trained in school. While this approach seems so simple and obvious, it is just not the way modern physicians are generally trained to think. This approach also requires that the clinician has a working knowledge of diet, vitamins, minerals, herbs, and other therapeutic interventions in addition to drugs and surgery since it favors the use of non-toxic and non-invasive interventions whenever possible. Most doctors are intrigued but yet intimidated by this approach because they feel like they were not trained in these matters and do not have the time or mechanisms to learn this information.

It should be stressed the *New Medicine* certainly does not reject what is miraculous and good about conventional medicine. The modern practitioners of this new medical approach, no matter what it is referred to by, embrace a collaborative relationship with all medical providers and stress an integrative approach to healthcare. It is obvious that conventional medical approaches are certainly necessary in acute illness, trauma, and end-stage disease, and in fact, excel in these circumstances. However, it is the chronically ill patients who cannot seem to get an accurate or definitive medical diagnosis from their standard medical providers that can benefit most from the *functional* approach. This new type of physician will often provide, or facilitate, through co-management, the blending of *alternative* and *conventional* approaches based on the appropriateness in each individual patient's situation.

If this approach to health care seems to make sense to you, and you would like to find a provider who is trained in this discipline, contact the *Institute for Functional Medicine* (www.functionalmedicine.org) for a list of trained providers in your area.

References:

1. Eisenberg DM, Davis RB, Ettner SL, Appel S, Wilkey S, Van Rompay M, et al. Trends in alternative medicine use in the United States, 1990-1997: results of a follow-up national survey. Jama. 1998 Nov 11;280(18):1569-75.

2. Lyon M. Healing the Hyperactive Brain Through the New Science of Functional Medicine. Calgary: Focused Publishing; 2000.

The Disorders

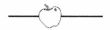

This section is meant to give you basic information on the use of vitamins, minerals, herbs, diet, and lifestyle modifications for some of the most common chronic health problems seen in the general population today. ***This information is not meant to be complete or exhaustive, nor is it meant to replace the advice and guidance of your doctor.*** For more detailed information, and a more complete list of disorders, please refer to the recommended, reader-friendly, books listed in the *Resources* section and marked with an asterisk (*). Remember, if you have not been properly diagnosed, or if your problem worsens, please see your healthcare professional immediately.

Disclaimer

This book is not meant to serve as medical advice and should not be interpreted to replace the necessity for diagnosis and direct management by a qualified healthcare provider.

ADHD (Attention Deficit Hyperactivity Disorder):

Supplementation:

Multivitamin-mineral; as directed on label

Vitamin B6 (P-5-P form preferred): 25-50 mg per day

Magnesium: 250-500 mg per day (magnesium-glycinate or bis-glycinate form preferred)

EPA-DHA: 500-1,000 mg per day

L-Tyrosine: 1,000 mg per day

L-Glutamine: 1,000 mg per day

5-Hydroxytryptophan (5-HTP): 50 mg per day

DMG (Dimethylglycine): 150 mg per day

Phosphatidyl Serine: 20 mg per day

American Ginseng (Panex quinquefolius): 100-200 mg per day (standard. to 55% ginsenosides)

Gingko biloba: 50-100 mg per day (standardized to 24% gingko flavone glycosides) Lactobacillus acidophilus: as directed on label

Since it is often difficult to get kids to swallow pills, particularly this many, a similar collection of nutrients has been combined with quality proteins, carbohydrates, and fats in a delicious meal replacement drink called *PediaFocus* (visit *healthyrevolutions.info* for information on this product). This product also contains a base of nutrients similar to a high-quality multivitamin-mineral supplement and can be used as a breakfast drink in order to assure that proper levels of critical nutrients are being consumed by the overactive child. This product can also be used by teenagers and adults as well.

Dietary Modifications:

The consumption of non-processed whole foods is critical in order to avoid chemical food additives as much as possible in these individuals. Simple sugars, including high-fructose corn syrup, should be limited as much as possible in the child's diet. An oligoantigenic diet (avoid gluten, dairy, corn, etc.) should be followed for several weeks followed by reintroduction of foods one at a time in order to determine if any of these specific foods contribute to a worsening of symptoms. Variation in food consumption patterns should be strived for. The guidance of a nutritionally-minded clinician is strongly advised to help guide you with these difficult dietary issues and to determine specific food allergens for your child by laboratory analysis (i.e. The *Comprehensive Metabolic Profile*).

Anxiety:

Supplementation:

GABA (Gamma-aminobutyric acid): 300 mg twice daily

Ashwaganda (Withania somnifera): 300 mg twice daily

Valerian Root (Valeriana officinalis): 300mg three times daily

Passion Flower (Passiflora incarnata): 300 mg three times daily

Magnesium: 250-500 mg per day (magnesium-glycinate or bis-glycinate form preferred)

Calcium: 150-300 mg per day (calcium malate, glycinate or citrate forms preferred)

Lifestyle Modifications:

1. Reduce your social and occupational stressors as much as possible

2. Keep predictable sleep patterns (in bed by 10 pm, don't over sleep in morning)

3. Get moderate exercise, but do not over-exercise

4. Try and get exposure to sunlight first thing in the morning

5. Engage in meditation, yoga, guided imagery, prayer, etc., on a regular basis

Arthritis:

Supplementation:

Degenerative (DJD):

Glucosamine sulfate: 500 mg three times per day

Chondroitin sulfate: 400 mg three times per day (optional)

Vitamin E (mixed): 400-800 IU per day

Vitamin C (with bioflavonoids): 1,000 mg three times per day

EPA-DHA: 1,000 mg three times per day

Rheumatoid:

Vitamin E (mixed): 400-800 IU per day

Vitamin C (with bioflavonoids): 1,000 mg three times per day

EPA-DHA: 1,000 mg three times per day

Tumeric (Curcuma longa): 300mg three times daily (standardized to 95% curcuminoids)

Ginger (Zingiber officinale): 200mg three times daily (standardized to 5% ginerols)

Boswellia (Boswellia serrata): 400mg three times daily (standardized to 70% boswellic acids)

Dietary Modifications:

Avoid foods containing inflammatory fatty acids, such as dairy products and commercially raised corn-fed beef and poultry. Use free-range meats if consumption of these foods is desired. Utilize flax seeds and monounsaturated fats in diet, such as extra virgin olive oil.

Lifestyle Modifications:

1. Engage in moderate non-weight bearing exercise (i.e. swimming, stationary bike, etc.) in order to maintain mobility

2. Rest affected joints during flare-ups

Bladder Infection:

Supplementation:

Vitamin C: 1,000 mg every four hours when symptomatic

Cranberry capsules: 3-4 every four hours when symptomatic

Garlic (Allium sativum): 2-3 capsules every four hours when symptomatic

Lactobacillus acidophilus: as directed on label

Dietary Modifications:

Liberal consumption of water is highly recommended. The drinking of natural (no sugar added) cranberry juice is also helpful (available at most health food stores). Avoid foods high in simple sugars. See your doctor if symptoms of burning or urgency worsen or if the infection does not clear within 2 days.

Colds and Flu:

Supplementation:

Vitamin C: 1,000 mg every four hours when symptomatic

Echinacea (Echinacea angustifolia or purpurea): 300 mg every four hours when symptomatic

Andrographis (Andrographis paniculata): 200-400 mg every four hours when symptomatic

Garlic (Allium sativum): 600 mg every four hours when

symptomatic

Zinc lozenges: 1 lozenge every 2-3 hours

Dietary Modifications:

1.   Drink plenty of fluids

2.   Avoid foods high in simple sugars

Lifestyle Modifications:

1.   Get plenty of rest

2.   No exercising while symptomatic

Constipation:

Supplementation:

Psyllium or other quality fiber supplement: 1 Tbsp three to four times per day with water

Lactobacillus acidophilus: as directed on label

Folic acid: 300 mcg two times per day

Magnesium: 250-500 mg two times per day

Dietary Modifications:

1.   Add more unrefined non-processed high-fiber foods to diet

2.   Drink plenty of fresh water

Depression (mild):

Supplementation:

5-Hydroxytryptophan (5-HTP): 50-100 mg per three times day

or

St. John's Wort (Hypericum perforatum): 450 mg two to three times per day

*(standardized to 0.3% hypericins)

Lifestyle Modifications:

1.   Keep predictable sleep patterns (in bed by 10 pm, don't over sleep in morning)

2.   Get moderate exercise, but do not over-exercise

3.   Engage in meditation, yoga, guided imagery, prayer, etc., on a regular basis

4.   Reduce your social and occupational stressors as much as possible

*If depression is moderate to severe and/or long-lasting, see a physician as soon as possible.

Diabetes:

Supplementation:

Chromium: 100 mcg three times per day (glycinate or bis-glycinate form preferred)

Vanadium: 10 mg three times per day (nicotinate-glycinate form preferred)

Magnesium: 200 mg three times per day (magnesium glycinate or bis-glycinate form preferred)

Vitamin E (mixed): 400-800 IU per day

Antioxidant formula: as directed on label

Vitamin C: 1,000 mg three times per day

B-Complex: 50 mg three times per day

EPA-DHA (Omega-3 fatty acids); 1,000 mg three times per day

L-Carnitine: 100 mg three times per day

Fenugreek (Trigonella foenum-graecum): 300 mg three times per day

Gymnema sylvestre: 100 mg three times per day

Cinnamon (Cinnamomum cassia / zeylanicum): 500 mg three times per day

Dietary Modifications:

1. Eat small, frequent meals instead of three large meals per day.

2. Eat a diet consisting of non-starchy, complex carbohydrates balanced with adequate lean protein, mono-unsaturated fats, and fiber (30-40 gm/day) (*See section on diet)

3. Eliminate or avoid: simple sugars and refined carbohydrates, fried foods, alcohol and tobacco. Dairy product avoidance is recommended in Type I diabetes.

Lifestyle Modifications:

1. Monitor blood glucose levels several times daily with home monitoring system. Alter diet in   order to stay within normal glucose parameters.

2.   Avoid obesity and strive to achieve ideal body weight in Type II Diabetes Mellitus.

3.   Exercise regularly.

Diarrhea:

Supplementation:

Lactobacillus acidophilus: as directed on label

Folic acid: 300 mcg two times per day

Psyllium or other quality fiber supplement: 1 Tbsp three to four times per day with water

Florastor (Saccharomyces boulardii lyo): 250 mg twice daily

B-Complex: 50 mg three times per day

Valerian Root (Valeriana officinalis): 200-300mg every four hours as needed

Chamomile tea: as needed

Dietary Modifications:

1.   Add more unrefined non-processed high fiber foods to diet

Fibromyalgia:

Supplementation:

Magnesium: 500-1,000 mg per day in divided dosages (glycinate or malate form preferred)

Malic Acid: 1,200-2,400mg per day in divided dosages

B-Complex: 50-100 mg three times per day

CoQ10: 100 mg twice daily

L-Carnitine: 500 mg two to three times daily

Manganese: 20mg per day in divided dosages....

Cordyceps mycelia (Cordyceps sinensis): 400-600 mg three times per day

5-Hydroxytryptophan (5-HTP): 50-100 mg per three times day (only under supervision)

Dietary Modifications:

1. Avoid food allergens and caffeine!

2. The consumption of non-processed whole foods is critical in order to avoid chemical food   additives as much as possible. Simple sugars should be limited as much as possible in the diet. An oligoantigenic diet (avoid gluten, dairy, corn, etc.) should be followed for several weeks followed by reintroduction of foods one at a time in order to determine if any of these specific foods contribute to a worsening of symptoms. Variation in food consumption patterns should be strived for. The guidance of a nutritionally-minded clinician is strongly advised to help guide you with these difficult dietary issues, and determine specific food allergens (consider taking the *Comprehensive Metabolic Profile* by visiting *healthyrevolution.info* to find a provider near you).

Lifestyle Modifications:

1. Keep predictable sleep patterns (in bed by 10 pm, don't over sleep in morning)

2. Get moderate exercise, but do not over-exercise

*   It is highly recommended that you see a wellness physician, preferably one trained in *Functional medicine*, in order to determine if you may have health issues such as anemia, toxicity, intestinal problems, hypothyroidism, adrenal fatigue, among others, that may be the prime reason for your symptoms (i.e. fatigue, tenderness, cognitive problems, etc.), rather than true classic fibromyalgia syndrome. Read more about fibromyalgia at ***www.drdavidbrady.com*** by selecting the *published articles by Dr. Brady* button on the left and selecting *fibromyalgia*.

High Blood Pressure:

Supplementation:

Magnesium: 500 mg three times per day (magnesium glycinate or bis-glycinate form preferred)

Calcium: 250 mg three times per day (calcium malate, glycinate or citrate forms preferred)

Potassium: 200 mg three times per day

Garlic (Allium sativum): 500mg three times per day

Hawthorne (Crataegus oxyacantha): 400-800 mg two to three times daily

Dietary Modifications:

Limit salt consumption. Do not add salt at the table or while cooking. Avoid processed foods and snack foods that are very high in sodium. Whole, fresh, non-processed foods are highly encouraged.

Lifestyle Modifications:

1. Avoid obesity and strive to achieve ideal body weight.

2. Exercise regularly.

High Cholesterol and Cardiovascular Disease Risk:

Supplementation:

Niacin: 1000 mg two times per day

Magnesium: 250-500 mg per day (magnesium glycinate form preferred)

Garlic (Allium sativum): 500mg three times per day

Chromium: 200 mcg per day (bis-glycinate or glycinate form preferred)

B-Complex: 100 mg twice daily

Tocotrienols: 100-200 mg in evening

Red Yeast Rice Extract (Monascus purpureus): 600 mg twice daily (only under supervision)

Guggul (Commiphora mukul): 200-400 mg three times daily

*(standardized to 10% guggulsterones)

CoQ10: 100 mg twice daily

Dietary Modifications:

1. Eat a diet consisting of non-starchy, complex carbohydrates balanced with adequate lean protein,

mono-unsaturated fats, and fiber (30-40 gm/day) (*See *Diet* chapter)

2. Eliminate or avoid: simple sugars, refined carbohydrates, fried foods, alcohol, and tobacco.

Lifestyle Modifications:

1. Avoid obesity and strive to achieve ideal body weight.

2. Exercise regularly.

3. Have blood cholesterol, triglycerides, HDL, LDL, hs-CRP, lipoprotein-a, homocysteine, and fibrinogen levels checked yearly.

Hypothyroidism:

Supplementation:

L-Tyrosine: 500 mg two times per day

Atlantic Sea Kelp (Iodine source): 150-200 mg per day (do not exceed this dosage!)

Multivitamin and mineral: as directed on label

Selenium: 50-100 mcg daily

B-Complex: 50-100 mg three times per day

* Read more about hypothyroidism at *www.drdavidbrady.com* by selecting the *published articles by Dr. Brady* button on the left and selecting *hypothyroidism*.

* See a physician if symptoms persist in order to be evaluated for possible need for hormone replacement therapy.

Inflammation (sprain/strains, sport injuries, etc.):

Supplementation:

Proteolytic Enzymes (trypsin, chymotrypsin, bromelin, etc.): 3-4 tablets four times per day in between meals (*Do not take if you have an ulcer!*)

Bioflavonoids (quercetin, resperidin, rutin, etc.): 200 mg mixed bioflavonoids every two hours during acute phase

Tumeric (Curcuma longa): 300mg every 2 hours while swollen (standard. to 95% curcuminoids)

Ginger (Zingiber officinale): 200mg every 2 hours while swollen (standard. to 5% ginerols)

Boswellia (Boswellia serrata): 400mg every 2 hours while swollen (standard. to 70% boswellic acids)

EPA-DHA: 1,000 mg three times per day

Dietary Modifications:

Avoid foods containing inflammatory fatty acids, such as dairy products and commercially raised corn-fed beef and poultry. Use free-range meats if these foods are desired. Utilize flax seeds and monounsaturated fats in diet, such as extra virgin olive oil.

Lifestyle Modifications:

1. Rest affected area

2. Apply ice to effected area for 20 minutes every two hours while swollen

3. Do not apply heat while swollen

Muscle Tightness & Spasm:

Supplementation:

Valerian Root (Valeriana officinalis): 200-300mg every four hours as needed

Passion Flower (Passiflora incarnata): 100-200mg every four hours as needed

Magnesium: 500 mg three times per day (magnesium glycinate or bis-glycinate form preferred)

Calcium: 250 mg three times per day (calcium malate, glycinate or citrate forms preferred)

Lifestyle Modifications:

1. Engage in meditation, yoga, guided imagery, prayer, etc., on a regular basis

2. Reduce your social and occupational stressors as much as possible

3. Get moderate exercise, but do not over-exercise

* Consider being evaluated by a chiropractic physician, physical therapist and/or a massage therapist if condition becomes chronic.

Stress & Adrenal Fatigue:

Supplementation:

American Ginseng (Panex quinquefolius): 100-200 mg per day (standard. to 55% ginsenosides)

Ashwaganda (Withania somnifera): 300 mg twice daily

Phosphatidyl Serine: 50-100 mg per day

Vitamin C: 1,000 mg three times per day

B-complex: 50-100 mg three times per day

Optional:

Valerian Root (Valeriana officinalis): 300mg three times daily

Passion Flower (Passiflora incarnata): 300 mg three times daily

Magnesium: 250-500 mg per day (magnesium-glycinate or bis-glycinate form preferred)

Calcium: 150-300 mg per day (calcium malate, glycinate or citrate forms preferred)

Dietary Modifications:

1. Avoid food allergens and caffeine

Lifestyle Modifications:

1. Keep predictable sleep patterns (in bed by 10 pm, don't over sleep in morning)

2. Get moderate exercise, but do not over-exercise

3. Try and get exposure to sunlight first thing in the morning

4. Engage in meditation, yoga, guided imagery, prayer, etc., on a regular basis

5. Reduce your social and occupational stressors as much as possible

---

General References:

1. Fairfield KM, Fletcher RH. Vitamins for chronic disease prevention in adults: scientific review. Jama. 2002 Jun 19;287(23):3116-26.

2. Groff J, Gropper S. Advanced Nutrition and Human Metabolism. 3rd ed. Stamford, CT: Wadsworth; 2000.

3. Marz R. Medical Nutrition from Marz. 2nd ed. Portland: Omni-Press; 1999.

4. Shils M, Shike M, Ross A. Modern Nutrition in Health and Disease. 10th ed. Baltimore: Lippicott Williams & Wilkins; 2006.

5. Werbach M, Murray M. Botanical Influences on Illness. Tarzana, CA: Third Line Press; 1994.

6. Bacom A. Incorporating Herbal Medicine Into Clinical Practice. Philadelphia: F.A. Davis; 2002.

7. Blumenthal M, Busse W. The Complete German Commission E Monographs: Therapeutic Guide to Herbal Medicines. 1st ed. Philadelphia: Lippincott Williams & Wilkins; 1998.

8. Chevallier A. Encylopedia of Herbal Medicine. London: Dorling Kindersley; 2000.

9. Fetrow C, Avila J. Professional's Handbook of Complimentary & Alternative Medicines. Springhouse, PA: Springhouse; 1999.

10. Pizzorno J, Murray M. Textbook of Natural Medicine. 2nd ed. Edinburgh: Churchill Livingstone; 1999.

Resources

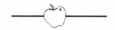

References and Suggested Texts

Books with the (*) before the title are suggested for the non-professional as basic, reader-friendly, resources for information on dietary, nutritional, herbal, and complimentary approaches to health and various disorders.

Diet Books Referenced:

Enter the Zone
Barry Sears, Ph.D.
Regan Books/HarperCollins
ISBN: 0-06-039150-2

Dr. Atkins' New Diet Revolution (3rd Edition)
Robert C. Atkins, M.D.
M. Evans Books
ISBN: 1-59-077002-3

Protein Power
Michael R. Eades, M.D.
Mary Dan Eades, M.D.
Bantam Books
ISBN: 0-55-357475-2

The New Sugar Busters
H. Leighton Steward
Morrison C. Bethea, M.D., et al.
Ballantine Books
ISBN: 0-34545-537-1

The South Beach Diet
Arthur Agaston, M.D.
Rodale, Inc.
ISBN: 0-157954-646-3

The Carbohydrate Addicts Diet
Richard F. Heller, M.D.
Rachael F. Heller, M.D.
Signet Publishers
ISBN: 0-45117-339-2

The Paleo Diet
Loren Cordain
Wiley Publishing
ISBN: 0-47126-755-4

New Pritikin Program
Robert Pritikin, M.D.
Pocket Books
ISBN: 0-67-173194-7

Eat More, Weight Less
Dean Ornish, M.D.
Harper Collins
ISBN: 0-06-095957-6

The MacDougal Program for Maximum Weight Loss
John A. McDougall, M.D.
Mary McDougall
Plume
ISBN: 0-45-227380-3

Eat Right for Your Type
Peter J. D'Adamo, N.D.
Catherine Whitney
Putnam Adult
ISBN: 0-399-14255-X

The 20-Day Rejuvenation Diet Program
Jeffrey S. Bland, Ph.D.
Sara H. Benum, M.A.
Keats Publishing
ISBN: 0-87983-760-8

Informational Books:

Textbook of Natural Medicine (3nd Ed)
Joseph E. Pizzorno, N.D.
Michael T. Murray, N.D.
Churchill Livingston
ISBN: 0-443-07300-7
(A complete and technical two-volume text for the nutritional practitioner)

Encyclopedia of Natural Medicine (2nd Ed)
Michael T. Murray, N.D.
Joseph E. Pizzorno, N.D.
Prima Publishing
ISBN: 0-7615-1157-1
(A more user-friendly and less technical work for the layperson)

Textbook of Nutritional Medicine
Melvyn R. Werbach, M.D.
Jeffrey Moss, D.D.S., C.N.S., C.C.N.
Third Line Press
ISBN: 0-9618550-9-6

Prescription for Nutritional Healing (3rd Edition)
James F. Balch, M.D.
Phyllis A. Balch, C.N.C.
Avery Publishing Group
ISBN: 1-58333-077-1

Prescription for Herbal Healing:
An Easy-to-Use A-Z Reference to Hundreds of Common Disorders and
Their Herbal Remedies
Phyllis A. Balch, C.N.C.
Robert Rister
Avery Publishing Group
ISBN: 0-8952-9869-4

Nutritional Influences on Illness (2nd Ed)
Melvyn R. Werbach, M.D.
Third Line Press
ISBN: 0-9618550-5-3

Botanical Influences on Illness (2nd Ed)
Melvyn R. Werbach, M.D.
Michael T. Murray, N.D.
Third Line Press
ISBN: 0-9618550-4-5

The Complete Illustrated Holistic Herbal
David Hoffman
Element Books
ISBN: 1-85230-758-7

The Professional's Handbook of Complimentary & Alternative Medicine
Charles W. Fetrow, PharmD
Juan R. Avila, PharmD
Springhouse
ISBN: 0-87434-971-0

The Nutrition Desk Reference
Robert H. Garrison, Jr., M.A., R.Ph
Elizabeth Somer, M.A., R.D.
Keats Publishing
ISBN: 0-87983-523-0

Power Healing
Leo Galland, M.D.
Random House
ISBN: 0-375-75139-4

Genetic Nutritioneering
Jeffrey S. Bland, Ph.D.
Sara H. Benum, M.A.
Keats Publishing
ISBN: 0-87983-921-X

Cracking the Metabolic Code
James B. LaValle, R.Ph., C.C.N.
Stacy Lundin Yale, R.N., B.S.N.
Basic Health Publications
ISBN: 1-59120-011-3

Instant Access to Chiropractic Guidelines and Protocols (2nd Edition)
Lew Huff, D.C.
David M. Brady, N.D., D.C., C.C.N., D.A.C.B.N.
Mosby
ISBN: 0-32303-068-8

The Chiropractic Profession
David Chapman-Smith
NCMIC Group, Inc.
ISBN: 1-892734-02-8

Organon of the Medical Art
Samuel Hahnemann, M.D. (H)
Birdcage Books
ISBN: 1-889613-01-0

Lectures on Homeopathic Philosophy
James Tyler Kent, M.D. (H)
North Atlantic Books
ISBN: 0-913028-61-4

Repertory of the Homeopathic Materia Medica
James Tyler Kent, M.D. (H)
B. Jain Publishers
ISBN: 81-7021-153-0

The Web That Has No Weaver:
Understanding Chinese Medicine
Ted Kapchuk, O.M.D.
Congdon & Weed, Inc.
ISBN: 0-86553-109-9

*Healing the Hyper Active Brain,
Through the New Science of Functional Medicine
Michael R. Lyon, M.D.
Focused Publishing
ISBN: 0-9685108-0-9

*Beyond Antibiotics,
50 (or so) Ways to Boost Immunity and Avoid Antibiotics
Michael A. Schmidt
Lendon H. Smith
Keith W. Sehnert
North Atlantic Books
ISBN: 1-55643-180-5

*The Cancer Industry
Ralph W. Moss
Paragon House
ISBN: 1-55778-075-7

*Don't Sweat The Small Stuff...and it's all small stuff
Richard Carlson, Ph.D.
Hyperion Publishing
ISBN: 0-7868-8185-2

*The Circadian Prescription: Get in Step with your Body's Natural Rhythms
Sidney M. Baker
Karen Baar
Putnam Adult
ISBN: 0-3991-4596-6

Resources and Organizations

David M. Brady, N.D., D.C., C.C.N., D.A.C.B.N.
www.drdavidbrady.com

*Resources for your doctor to acquire training in functional and complimentary medicine. Dr. Brady does NOT offer clinical telephone consultations directly with patients. However, Dr. Brady does maintain a private practice in Orange, CT at 203-799-7733 where he does accept new patients. For information on the **Comprehensive Metabolic Profile** and unique supplement programs to meet your foundational nutritional needs please visit **HealthRevolution.info** to find a practitioner near you.

The Institute for Functional Medicine
P.O. Box 1729
Gig Harbor, WA 98335
800-228-0622
www.functionalmedicine.org

The American Association of Naturopathic Physicians
4435 Wisconsin Ave NW, Suite 403
Washington, DC 20016
866-538-2267
www.naturopathic.org

The American College for Advancement in Medicine
23121 Verdugo Drive, Suite 204
Laguna Hills, CA 92653
949-583-7666
www.acam.org

International College of Integrative Medicine
707 Stanbridge St.
Norristown, PA 19401
866-464-5226
www.icimed.com

The American Academy of Environmental Medicine
7701 East Kellogg, Suite 625
Wichita, Kansas 67207
316-684-5500
www.aaem.com

American Clinical Board of Nutrition
6855 Browntown Road
Front Royal, VA 22630
540-635-8844
www.acbn.org

The International & American Association of Clinical Nutritionists
15280 Addison Road, Ste. 130
Addison, TX 75001
972-407-9089
www.iaacn.org

Clinical Nutrition Certification Board
5200 Keller Springs Road, Suite 410
Dallas, Texas 75248
972-250-2829
www.cncb.org

Certification Board for Nutrition Specialists
& The American College of Nutrition
300 S. Duncan Ave., Ste. 225
Clearwater, FL 33755
727-466-6068
www.amcollnutr.org

The American Chiropractic Association
1701 Clarendon Blvd.
Arlington, VA 22209
800-986-4636
www.amerchiro.org

The American Herbalists Guild
1931 Gaddis Road
Canton, GA 30115
770-751-6021
www.healthy.net/herbalists

The North American Society of Homeopaths
11222 East Pike Street, #1122
Seattle, WA 98122
206-720-7000
www.homeopathy.org

The American Association of Oriental Medicine
433 Front Street
Catasauqua, PA 18032
610-266-1433
www.aaom.org

Cancer Decisions.com & The Moss Report
Ralph W. Moss, Ph.D.
144 St. John's Place
Brooklyn, NY 11217
718-636-4433
www.cancerdecisions.com

X-iser
P.O. Box 406
Selersville, PA 18960
617-510-6355
www.healthyrevolution.info

Four-Year Colleges of Naturopathic Medicine
*The naturopathic medical schools listed below are the only programs to have been granted accreditation or candidacy-status for accreditation by the Council on Naturopathic Medical Education (CNME) and produce graduates who are eligible to sit the Naturopathic Physician Licensing Examinations (NPLEX) to qualify for official licensure as naturopathic physicians in states with enacted naturopathic legislation.

•   Bastyr University, College of Naturopathic Medicine (Bothel, WA)

- National College of Naturopathic Medicine (Portland, OR)
- Southwest College of Naturopathic Medicine (Phoenix, AZ)
- The University of Bridgeport, College of Naturopathic Medicine (Bridgeport, CT)
- Canadian College of Naturopathic Medicine (Toronto, Ontario, Canada)
- Boucher Institute of Naturopathic Medicine (New Westminster, BC, Canada)

States, Territories and Provinces with Licensure or Registration for Naturopathic Physicians

- Alaska
- Arizona
- California
- Connecticut
- District of Columbia
- Hawaii
- Idaho
- Kansas
- Maine
- Montana
- New Hampshire
- Oregon
- Utah
- Vermont
- Washington
- US Territories: Puerto Rico and Virgin Islands
- Canadian Provinces

Federally Recognized Academic Accrediting Bodies:

The following are the six federally recognized regional general institutional accrediting bodies in the United States:

North Central Association of Colleges and Schools, The Higher Learning Commission: degree-granting institutions of higher education in Arizona, Arkansas, Colorado, Illinois, Indiana, Iowa, Kansas, Michigan, Minnesota, Missouri, Nebraska, New Mexico, North Dakota, Ohio, Oklahoma, South Dakota, West Virginia, Wisconsin, and Wyoming, including schools of the Navajo Nation and the accreditation of programs offered via distance education within these institutions.

Middle States Association of Colleges and Schools, Commission on Higher Education: institutions of higher education in Delaware, the District of Columbia, Maryland, New Jersey, New York, Pennsylvania, Puerto Rico, and the U.S. Virgin Islands, including distance education programs offered at those institutions.

New England Association of Schools and Colleges, Commission on Institutions of Higher Education: institutions of higher education in Connecticut, Maine, Massachusetts, New Hampshire, Rhode Island, and Vermont that award bachelors, masters, and/or doctoral degrees and associate degree-granting institutions in those states that include degrees in liberal arts or general studies among their offerings, including the accreditation of programs offered via distance education within these institutions.

Northwest Commission on Colleges and Universities: postsecondary educational institutions in Alaska, Idaho, Montana, Nevada, Oregon, Utah, and Washington and the accreditation of such programs offered via distance education within these institutions.

Southern Association of Colleges and Schools, Commission on Colleges: degree-granting institutions of higher education in Alabama, Florida, Georgia, Kentucky, Louisiana, Mississippi, North Carolina, South Carolina, Tennessee, Texas, and Virginia, including distance education programs offered at those institutions.

Index

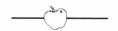

A

academic accrediting bodies, *191*
    North Central Association of Colleges and Schools, *191*
    Middle States Association of Colleges and Schools, *191*
    New England Association of Schools and Colleges, *191*
    Northwest Commission on Colleges and Universities, *191*
    Southern Association of Colleges and Schools, *191*
acid(s),
    amino acid, *36, 57, 126, 148*
        - metabolism of, *27*
    Arachadonic, *23, 24, 25*
    ascorbic acid, *52*
    caffeic acid, *78*
    essential fatty acids, *53, 60*
    gamma-aminobutyric acid (GABA), *94, 165*
    hydrogenated trans-fatty acids, *23, 33*
    omega-6 fatty acids, *53*
    omega-3 fatty acids, *20, 53, 171*
    valerenic acid, *94, 95*
Acupuncturist, *148, 151, 152, 156*
Agaston, Arthur, M.D., *34, 182*
Alkaloids, *66, 80, 88, 90, 94*
Allopathic, *1, 2, 127, 129, 130, 132, 133, 160*

Alzheimer's Disease, *18, 55, 85, 111, 120*
American Academy of Environmental Medicine, The, 188
American Association of Naturopathic Physicians, The, 187
American Association of Oriental Medicine, The, 189
American Chiropractic Association, The, 188
American Clinical Board of Nutrition, The, xi, 134, 188
American College for Advancement in Medicine, The, 128, 187
American Herbalists Guild, The, 143, 189
American Dietetic Association, 14
anti-,
    bacterial, *89*
    carcinogenic, *16, 23*
    coagulatory, *85*
    emetic, *83*
    fungal, *78, 81, 89*
    neoplastic (cancer), *78*
    oxidant, *16, 17, 20, 23, 30, 31, 53, 55, 56, 57, 60, 83, 84,*
    85, 121, 123, 124, 170
    viral, *78*
Atherosclerosis Regression Study, *44*
Atkins, Robert C., M.D., *181*
attention deficit hyperactivity disorder (ADHD), *61, 111, 164*
autoimmune and chronic inflammatory diseases, *20*
    Alzheimer's, *18, 55, 85, 111, 120*
    Celiac, *18, 35*
    Grave's Disease, *19*
    Hashimoto's Thyroiditis, *19, 36*
    Lupus, *24, 79*
    multiple sclerosis, *24, 79*
    Parkinson's disease, *18, 55, 111*
    pre-diabetes, *24*
    rheumatoid arthritis, *24, 83*
Avila, Juan R., PharmD *97, 180, 184*

B

Baar, Karen, *36, 108, 186*
Baker, Sidney M., *28, 36, 108, 186*
Balsch, James F., M.D., *49*
Balsch, Phyllis A., C.N.C., *49*
basic therapeutic nutritional protocols, *49*
Benum, Sara H., M.A., *183, 185*
Berberis,
    aquifolium (Oregon grape, mahonia), *88*
    vulgaris (barberry), *88*
beta-carotene, *55, 56, 60*
Bethea, Morrison C., M.D., et al., *10, 35, 182*
*Beyond Antibiotics, 50 (or so) Ways to Boost Immunity and
    Avoid Antibiotics, 186*
Biochemistry, *11, 28, 51, 55, 121, 142, 157*
black cohosh, *76, 77*
    Actaea racemosa, *76*
    Cimicifuga racemosa, *76*
    black snakeroot, *76*
    bugbane, *76*
    mugwort, *76*
    cimicifuga, *76*
    macrotys, *76*
    rattleroot, *76*
    rattleweed, *76*
    sqaw root, *76*
Bland, Jeffrey S., Ph.D., *183, 185*
Botanical Influences on Illness (2nd Ed), 97, 180, 184
botanical medicines, *65*
Brady, David M. N.D., D.C., C.C.N., D.A.C.B.N., *xi, 185, 187*

C

Calcium, *55, 56, 60, 91, 155, 166, 174, 178, 179,*
    calcium-glycinate, *54*
    calcium-malate, *54*
    calcium-citrate, *55*
    coral-calcium, *55*
    calcium-carbonate, *55*
Cambridge Heart Antioxidant Study, *44, 61, 62*
CancerDecisions.com, 189
Cancer Industry, The, 186
cardiovascular disease, *36, 44, 55, 56, 62, 118, 125, 175*
Carlson, Richard, PhD, *106, 186*
Celiac, *18, 35*
Certification Board for Nutrition Specialists & The American College of Nutrition, 188
Chapman-Smith, David, *185*
Chiropractic, *xi, 49, 127, 130, 131, 132, 133, 134, 140, 151, 154, 155, 158, 160, 178, 188*
Chiropractic Profession, The, 185
Chlorine, *29, 111*
cholesterol, high, *8, 10, 175*
Chromium *56, 60, 170, 175*
    chromium-glycinate, *56*
    chromium bis-glycinate, *56*
Circadian Prescription: Get in Step with your Body's Natural Rhythms, The, 28, 36, 108, 186
circadian rhythms, *27*
Clinical Nutrition Certification Board, 188
Co-enzyme Q10 (ubiquinone), *56*
Collagen, *52*
Colleges of Naturopathic Medicine, Four Year, *xi, 189*
Complete Illustrated Holistic Herbal, The, 184

complex carbohydrate, *8, 10, 17, 171, 175*
complimentary, *16, 65, 90, 97, 128, 148, 157, 180, 181, 187*
Comprehensive Metabolic Profile, *32, 33, 57, 60, 105, 122, 124, 125, 165, 173, 187*
Coptis chinensis (goldthread), *88*
Cordain, Loren, Ph.D., *7, 17, 36, 182*
Cracking the Metabolic Code, 185
crisis-centered medical model, *4*

D

D'Adamo, Peter J., N.D., *7, 183*
d-alpha-tocopherol, *44*
depression, *4, 51, 77, 85, 91, 92, 93, 96, 119, 169, 170*
detoxification, *26, 61, 122*
DGLA, *54*
DHA, *54, 164, 166, 167, 171, 177*
Diabetes, *2, 8, 10, 14, 17 19, 24, 26, 34, 35, 36, 56, 81, 99, 103, 170, 171, 172*
Diet,
    20-Day Rejuvenation Diet Program, The, 183
    Carbohydrate Addict's Diet, The, 10
    Circadian Prescription, The, 28, 36, 108, 186
    Dr. Atkin's New Diet Revolution, 7, 10, 34,181
    Eat More, Weigh Less, 7
    Eat Right 4 Your Type, 183
    McDougall Program, The, 7
    New Pritikin Program, The, 7, 34, 182
    Paleo Diet, The, 7, 17, 34, 182
    Protein Power Diet, The, 10, 35, 181
    South Beach Diet, The, 7, 13. 34,182
    Standard American Diet (S.A.D.), *10, 19, 28*

Sugar Busters, 10, 35, 182
   Zone, The, 7, 13, 16, 20, 34, 181
dietary guidelines, *8, 14, 20, 33*
Dietician, *14, 17, 147, 148*
Don't Sweat the Small Stuff.....and it's all Small Stuff, 106, 186

E

Eades, Mary Dan, M.D., *10, 35, 181*
Eades, Michael R., M.D. *35, 181*
Echinacea, *68, 70, 71, 78, 79, 168*
   Angustifolia, *78, 168*
   Purpurea, *78, 168*
   Pallida, *78*
   Encapsulated, *72*
   Tableted, *72*
Ecosanoids, *81*
Encyclopedia of Natural Medicine (2nd Ed), 49, 183
Entering the Zone, 13
Environmental Protection Agency (EPA), *111, 112*
Enzymes, *30, 51, 55, 177*
Ephedra, *79*
   Ephedra sinica, *79*
   Ephedra nevadensis, *79*
   Ma Huang, *79*
   Chinese ephedra, *79*
   desert tea, *79*
   Brigham tea, *79*
   Mexican tea, *79*
   Mormon tea, *79*
Ephedrine, *80*
   Pseudoephedrine, *80, 81*
   nor-pseudoephedrinem, *80*

erectile dysfunction, *85*
Esoteric and Intuitive Healers, *155, 156*
essential oils, *78*

F

fat soluble vitamins, *25*
fats, *8, 9, 10, 12, 13, 16, 20, 23, 24, 25, 33, 54, 57, 90, 121, 123, 164, 167, 171, 176, 177*
    monosaturated fats, *20*
    polyunsaturated fats, *20*
fatty acids, *20, 23, 33, 34, 53, 60, 123, 167, 171, 177*
    essential, *53, 60*
    omega-6 fatty acids, *53*
    omega-3 fatty acids, *20, 53, 171*
Federal Drug Administration (FDA), *46, 80*
Fibromyalgia, *2, 107, 172, 174*
fish oil, *53*
flavonoids, *78, 84, 85, 86, 91, 94*
fluorine, *28*
food pyramid, *14*
Framingham Study, 8
free radicals, *53, 55, 123*
free-range, *19, 24, 25, 167, 177*
Fetrow, Charles W. PharmD, *184*

G

Galland, Leo, M.D. , *184*
gamma-aminobutyric acid (GABA), *92, 94, 165*
garlic (allium sativum), *81, 82, 84. 86, 168, 174, 175*
Garrison, Robert H. Jr., M.A., R.Ph., *184*

Genetic Nutritioneering, 185
genetic polymorphism, *8*
genetically altered products, *22*
Ginger, *82, 83, 84, 86, 167, 177*
    Zingiber officinale, *82*
    Gingerols, *83, 84*
    Zingiberol, *83*
    Curcumene, *83*
    zingibain, *83*
Ginkgo, *84, 85, 86, 87*
    Ginkgo biloba, *84*
    Maidenhair, *84*
    Kew tree, *84*
Ginseng, *86, 87, 88, 164, 178*
    Panex ginseng/quinquefolium, *86*
    Chinese, *86*
    Korean, *86*
    Panex quinquefolium (American ginseng) , *86*
    Eleutherococcussenticosus (Siberian ginseng) , *86*
GLA, *54*
glycemic index, *19*
Goldenseal, *88, 89, 90*
    Hydrastis Canadensis, *88, 90*
    eye root, *88*
    eye balm, *88*
    yellow root, *88*
    Indian turmeric, *88*
    jaundice root, *88*
grass fed, *19, 24*
Grave's Disease, *19*

H

Hahnemann, Samuel M.D. (H), *145, 158, 185*

Hashimoto's Thyroiditis, *19, 36*

Healing the Hyper Active Brain Through the New Science of Functional Medicine, 160, 186

Health Professional's Follow-up Study, *44*

Heller, Rachael F., M.D., *10, 35, 182*

Heller, Richard F., M.D., *10, 35, 182*

Herbalists, *71, 75, 89, 130, 139, 140, 141, 142, 143, 152*

herbs, forms of, *5, 46, 47-49, 57, 60, 65-69, 70-74, 76, 86, 130, 131, 136, 139, 143, 161*

    dry powders, *72*

    liquid extracts, *72, 73*

    solid extracts, *72, 73*

    decoctions, *72, 73*

    effusions, *72, 73*

    raw herb, *72, 74*

    standardized, *58, 70, 72, 75, 86, 141*

    non-standardized, *72, 73, 74*

    reductionist, *75, 149*

    Ayrevadic, *75*

High Density Lipid ("good" cholesterol or HDL), *31, 56, 176*

Hoffman, David, *184*

Homeopathic, *131, 143, 144, 145, 146, 147, 158, 185*

hormonal biorhythms, *27*

Huff, Lew, D.C., *185*

human genome, *18*

hydrastine, *88*

hydrogenated, *9, 23, 24, 33*

hypericum perforatum, *91, 170*

    see also St. John's Wort

hypothyroid, *41, 174, 176*

I

Instant Access to Chiropractic Guidelines and Protocols (2nd Edition), 185
Institute for Functional Medicine, The, 129, 162, 187
International & American Association of Clinical Nutritionists, The, 188
International College of Integrative Medicine, 128, 187
iodine deficient, *41*

K

Kapchuk, Ted O.M.D., *186*
Ketogenic, *11, 12*
Ketones, *12, 13*
Ketostix, *12*
Kent, James Tyler M.D. (H), *146, 185*

L

LaValle, James B. R.Ph., C.C.N., *185*
L-Carnitine, *57, 60, 171, 173*
L-Glutathione, *57, 60*
Lectures on Homeopathic Philosophy, 146, 158, 185
Leighton-Steward, H., *10, 182*
lipid peroxidation, *53*
liver, *30, 46, 56, 76, 87, 88, 90, 95, 132, 148, 155*
    degeneration of the, *30*
    cirrhosis of the, *30*
    failure, *30*
Low Density Lipid ("bad" cholesterol or LDL), *31, 176*
Lupus Erythematosus, *24, 79*
Lyon, Michael M.D., *160, 161, 162, 186*

M

macular degeneration, *85*

magnesium, *26, 55, 164, 166, 169, 172, 174, 175, 178, 179*
  magnesium-glycinate, *55, 164, 166, 179*
  magnesium-malate, *55*

Massage Therapists, *153, 154, 155, 156*

McDougall, John, M.D., *182*

McDougall, Mary, *182*

medical disciplines and philosophies,
  Acupuncturist, *148, 151, 152, 156*
  Allopathic, *1, 2, 127, 129, 130, 132, 133, 160*
  Chiropractic, *49, 127, 130, 131, 132, 133, 134, 140, 151, 154, 155, 158, 160, 178, 188*
  Dietician, *14, 17, 147, 148*
  Esoteric and Intuitive Healers, *155, 156*
  Herbalists , *71, 75, 89, 130, 139, 140, 141, 142, 143, 152*
  Homeopathic, *131, 143, 144, 145, 146, 147, 158, 185*
  Massage Therapists, *153, 154, 155, 156*
  Naturopathic, *xi, 49, 70, 75, 133, 135-138, 140, 142-143, 155, 189, 190*
  Nutritionist, *9, 13, 18, 27, 50, 116, 124, 139, 147, 148, 188*
  Oriental Medicine, *86, 87, 148, 149, 150, 151, 152, 189*
  Osteopathic, *127, 128, 129, 130, 155*

Metabolic Profiling, *32, 33, 54, 57, 60, 105, 122, 124, 125, 165, 173, 187*

Metabolism, *11, 51, 119, 126*

Moss, Jeffrey, D.D.S., C.N.S., C.C.N., *ix, 183*

Moss, Ralph W., Pd.D., *189*

Moss Report, The, 189

Multiple Sclerosis, *24, 79*

multi-specialty integrative medicine, *5*

Murray, Michael T., N.D., *183, 184*

N

National Institutes of Health (NIH), *46*

Naturopathic, *xi, 49, 70, 75, 133, 135-138, 140, 142-143, 155, 189, 190*

Naturopathic Physicians, licensure or registration of, *136, 189, 190*

neurological degeneration, *30*

North American Society of Homeopaths, The, 189

Nurse's Health Study, *44*

Nutrition Desk Reference, The, 184

Nutritional Influences on Illness (2nd Edition), 63, 84

Nutritionist, *9, 13, 18, 27, 50, 116, 124, 139, 147, 148, 188*

O

Organic, *19, 22, 25, 113, 116, 122, 125, 126*

Organon of the Medical Art, 158, 185

Orgenon of the Healing Art, The, 146

Oriental Medicine, *86, 87, 148, 149, 150, 151, 152, 189*

Ornish, Dean, M.D, *34, 182*

P

Parkinson's disease, *18, 55, 111*

Peptide, *57*

peripheral vascular disease, *85*

pesticide, *113*

    residues, *22, 111*

    toxins, *22*

pharmacological, *48*

phytonutrients, *16, 23*

Pizzorno, Joseph E., N.D., *49, 97, 183*

premenstrual syndrome (PMS), *85*
Prescription for Nutritional Healing (3rd Edition), 183
*Prescription for Herbal Healing: An Easy-to-Use A-Z
    Reference, 184*
proprietary prescription drugs, *45*
polymorphism, genetic, *8*
polysaccharides, *78*
Power Healing, 184
Pre-diabetes, *24*
Pritikin, Robert, M.D., *10, 182*
*Professional's Handbook of Complimentary & Alternative
    Medicine, The, 97, 180, 184*
Prostaglandins, *83*

R

Recommended Daily Allowances (RDA), *50*
Recommended Daily Intakes (RDI), *50*
Repertory of the Homeopathic Materia Medica, 185
rheumatoid arthritis, *24, 83*
Rister, Robert, *184*

S

saturated animal fats, *8, 9, 23, 33*
Schmidt, Michael A., *186*
science foods, *21, 24*
Sears, Barry, Ph.D., *7, 13, 14, 16, 34, 181*
Sehnert, Keith W., *186*
Selenium, *55, 176*
Selye, Hans, M.D., *102*

Smith, Lendon H., *186*

St. John's Wort, *71, 91, 92, 93, 96, 170*

    Hypericum perforatum, *91, 170*

    Klamath weed, *91*

    Devil's scourge, *91*

Stress, *7, 30, 87, 92, 100, 102, 103, 104, 105, 106, 107, 108, 113, 117, 121*

Stroke, *18, 31, 53, 80, 82, 85, 123*

Sodium, *55, 174*

Somer, Elizabeth, M.A., R.D., *184*

synthetic compound, *46*

T

Textbook of Nutritional Medicine, 63, 183

therapeutic application, *46*

thyroid goiters, *41*

Tiller, William Ph.D., *145*

tinitis (ringing of the ear), *85*

tocopherols, *53*

    alpha tocopherols, *44, 53, 61*

    beta tocopherols, *53*

    gamma tocopherols, *53*

    delta tocopherols, *53*

toxicity, *30, 67, 82, 111, 123, 174*

trans-fats, *9, 24*

U

Understanding Chinese Medicine, 186

V

valerian root, *67, 94, 165, 172, 178, 179*
  valeriana officinalis, *94, 165, 172, 178, 179*
vitamin,
  - C, *39, 50, 51, 52, 55, 60, 104, 166, 167, 168, 171, 177*
  - E, *39, 43, 44, 53, 55, 60, 61, 62, 166, 167, 170*

W

Werbach, Melvyn R., M.D., *63, 97, 180, 183, 184*
Whitney, Catherine, *183*
World Health Organization, *66, 139*

X

X-iser, 101, 189

Y

Yale, Stacy Lundin, R.N., B.S.N., *185*

Printed in the United States
203124BV00002B/424-495/A